AYURVEDA

THE A-Z GUIDE TO HEALING TECHNIQUES FROM ANCIENT INDIA

DR. HELEN MARY THOMAS

Dr. Helen Mary Thomas is Doctor of Chiropractic who has studied Ayurveda since 1987 with Dr. Deepak Chopra, Vasant Lad, Raju and especially her mentor, Dr. Narendra Pendse, MD of Pune and Mumbai, India. Dr. Helen Thomas and her husband Dr. Craig Thomas have established the Thomas Chiropractic Center in Santa Rosa, California. The center provides comprehensive and holistic techniques that synthesize chiropractic, Ayurveda, NAET, Bodyword, and Bioenergetics.

Dr. Thomas lectures frequently to public and professional audiences.

Dr. Thomas is available for individual consultations in her Santa Rosa office by calling 707-527-7313. She is available for telephone consultations and Vedic Astrology readings through her scheduling website, www.AskTheAyurvedaExpert.com.

More information is available through the following websites:

www.AyurvedaTeatmentGuide.com

www.ThomasAyurveda.com

www.IndigestionGuru.com

AYURVEDA
THE A-Z GUIDE
TO HEALING TECHNIQUES FROM
ANCIENT INDIA

Dr. Helen Mary Thomas, D. C.

Second Print Edition

© Copyright 2013 - Helen Mary Thomas

Santa Rosa, California, U.S.A.

Print Edition, License Notes

TABLE OF CONTENTS

CONTENTS

CONTENTS

PART TWO
THE A-Z GUIDE TO COMMON CONDITIONS AND
HOW TO TREAT THEM WITH AYURVEDA 137

iv

CONTENTS

I dedicate this book to my husband Craig for his eternal love and support of my efforts, and to my children, Margaret and Matthew, for sharing me with Ayurveda. I would like to acknowledge my teachers: my first and most endearing, my mother Margaret O'Connell-Skondin; my spiritual teachers, Baba Bhagawan Ramji and Harihar Ramji; and my Ayurvedic teachers Deepak Chopra, Vasant Lad, and many others. My profound, deepest thanks go to Drs. Narendra and Aruna Pendse for teaching me the profound and practical gift of clinical Ayurveda.

—Dr. Helen Mary Thomas

THE A-Z GUIDE

INTRODUCTION

- Dr. Helen Mary Thomas, D.C. -

"When I first came to Dr. Helen Thomas, I was feeling completely out of control—I felt like I'd never be able to catch up . . . exhausted, unfocused, pushing hard to make my business a success and pay the mortgage, recovering from a separation. I knew I was just about to hit the wall, and was concerned about my family history of diabetes and cancer. Although I was initially skeptical and cautious, I began light therapy, music therapy, aromatherapy, and an Ayurvedic eating pattern. Within five days things began to change. I could feel my energy shift. I am happier, more focused, and more balanced than I have ever been."

"During the past year I've taken off fifteen pounds without dieting or counting calories. By following an Ayurvedic program, I found that my energy became balanced, and the excess weight just fell off."

Whether you're interested in preventing serious disease and improving your health in general or you want to treat specific symptoms such as headache, overweight, or insomnia, Ayurveda works. These are just two examples of the many patients I have seen whose lives have changed thanks to Ayurveda. They are joined by thousands of other people all over the world who are living proof that this holistic, integrated health system is as effective as it was when it originated in India nearly six thousand years ago. Today the ancient beauty and wisdom of Ayurveda is spreading to the Western world, thanks in part to the success of the best-selling books and videotapes of Dr. Deepak Chopra, who was one of my teachers. The message of Ayurveda is falling on eager ears for good

AYURVEDA

reason: Although modern mainstream medicine has achieved enormous success in some areas, particularly traumatic injury, acute infections, and certain types of cancers, the track record is not so impressive for treating chronic diseases such as arthritis, multiple sclerosis, heart disease, and most types of cancer. Nor is conventional medicine known for its warm, caring, individualized treatment, or its ability to prevent disease in the first place.

Complementary, alternative, or unconventional therapies such as Ayurveda have stepped in to fill the gap, so much so that they are being called "the hidden mainstream." This phenomenon was recently documented in the New England Journal of Medicine when it published a survey that found that one out of three people used at least one unconventional therapy in 1990. Based on the survey results, the authors estimated that people actually make more visits to unconventional-therapy practitioners than to mainstream primary-care physicians, and are spending approximately the same total amount of money out-of-pocket ($10 billion) for unconventional therapies as for hospitalizations.

Ayurveda, a Sanskrit word that means "knowledge of life and longevity," is based on principles and rhythms found in nature. It makes use of daily and seasonal lifestyle practices (including diet, yoga, and meditation), healing herbs, purification therapies, and a life-affirming mental attitude. Although at first glance some Ayurvedic practices may seem exotic, foreign, or downright old-fashioned, they are in actuality universal, timeless, and as useful now as they were thousands of years ago. In my practice I have found that Ayurveda is more relevant than ever, since it seeks to restore harmony and balance in a world that is growing increasingly out of kilter, with pollution, stress, junk food, accelerating schedules, sedentary occupations, and passive pastimes.

When I came to Ayurveda in 1987, I had been a chiropractor for five years. In chiropractic I had a very specific tool, one that realigned the spine and opened up the circulation to enhance the healing wisdom of the body. Although this was helpful for my patients, for many people relief was temporary and they suffered from stubborn, recurrent

THE A-Z GUIDE

musculoskeletal pain. This troubled me as a professional and I looked for a way to go beyond the simple chiropractic adjustment. I had a personal interest too: Although I had been meditating for many years, and was able to keep up a busy practice while raising a family, I had to admit I was frequently exhausted.

When I discovered Ayurveda, I saw that this holistic approach could be the answer. I was easily able to combine chiropractic with Ayurveda, since Ayurveda had a tradition of spinal manipulation as part of a larger, more comprehensive model of health care. As a result of studying Ayurveda, I have learned how to understand people in a deep and profound way. Many of my patients have been moved to tears because until they were analyzed according to Ayurveda, no one understood them so deeply, and no one was able to help them understand themselves so profoundly.

Since 1987 I have used Ayurveda to bring thousands of patients to optimum levels of physical, psychological, and spiritual health. This multidimensionality is the missing link that Ayurveda provides, and that is of utmost importance from the Ayurvedic perspective. I have found that even people who exercise regularly, eat a "well-balanced" low-fat diet, and take vitamin supplements still get sick. In spite of their efforts something is still missing—they are not paying attention to their inner lives of mind and spirit and are out of sync with their own rhythms and the universal rhythms of nature. They lack connection and deep understanding of their inner selves and their outer world.

Daily Ayurvedic practices nurture the whole person and provide tools to make those connections. The body's natural rhythms and physiology are attended to, enabling you to better understand yourself and your place in the world and bringing you to a state of gentle pleasure, a blissful feeling of unity with the wholeness of the universe. You are in balance, and symptoms and sickness—the signs of imbalance--melt away. One of my patients expresses the benefits of Ayurveda this way:

AYURVEDA

"Ayurveda has brought me a greater sense of my connection with my body and has opened the door to a greater understanding of what being healthy really means—a balance of body, mind, and spirit."

Ayurveda has a mystical past, but remains a practical approach to everyday health. Supremely suitable for self-care, the Ayurvedic approach can help you cope with and perhaps redefine modern life. In the face of daily onslaughts, it can help you reestablish and maintain your overall equilibrium as well as treat specific symptoms—from allergies and acne to headache, insomnia, tension and anxiety, fatigue, indigestion, sexual problems, and hot flashes. Ayurveda can help you kick the coffee habit and start the day full of energy, yet calm and focused; achieve your ideal weight; relax without drugs; prevent premature aging and serious disease; manage stress and detoxify your mind and body; and gently and naturally channel the healing power of all five of your senses rather than artificially dull them or over-stimulate them.

Despite its growing popularity, books about Ayurveda tend to be more philosophical and complicated than they are practical. As an educator I have long wanted to be able to reach a wider audience than I can reach in my practice and lectures. In this book I have combined our experiences and abilities to present Ayurveda in a clear, streamlined, useful form. I will show you how to integrate Ayurveda into your everyday life and use it safely and effectively to take care of yourself. The book is divided into two parts. In Part One I provide you with a basic understanding of Ayurveda, and in Part Two I show you how Ayurveda can be used to treat specific emotional and physical troubles.

Part One consists of six chapters. Chapter 1 gives you the background, history, and fundamentals of the Ayurvedic philosophy of health and disease. Chapter 2 explains the three "doshas" that are the overall guide in tailoring Ayurvedic practices to the individual. It includes two self-assessments. The first will help you uncover the particular imbalances you are experiencing at this time so that they can be corrected with the Ayurvedic tools and practices described in the following chapters; the

THE A-Z GUIDE

second is to enable you to determine your essential nature so that you can learn how to support it Ayurvedically and maintain health and well-being once your symptoms have cleared up. Chapter 3 teaches you how to perform the fundamental practices of Ayurveda geared toward disease prevention, rejuvenation of all your organ systems, longevity and anti-aging, and spiritual and mental health. Chapter 4 contains instructions for assembling and using the herbs, spices, and food-based remedies that form a natural "medicine cabinet" for maintaining health as well as for treating specific health problems. According to Ayurveda, smell, sight, taste, hearing, and touch are the doorways to your internal physiology and thus are potent healing mechanisms. Chapter 5 shows you simple, enjoyable practices that you can use at home to take advantage of the healing capabilities of your five senses. In Chapter 6 I show you how the practices explained in previous chapters can fit into a daily and seasonal routine that is tailored specifically to you as an individual.

Part Two is a guide to more than sixty common conditions, arranged in easy-to-use A—Z format, along with simple steps for treating them Ayurvedically. Under each condition you will find a description from the Ayurvedic point of view, followed by specific herbal remedies and other techniques to incorporate into your daily lifestyle routine to help restore balance and health naturally.

You'll also find books and other informational resources we recommend if you wish to deepen your knowledge and practice of Ayurveda.

Ayurveda is a complete and holistic system that recognizes that each person is a unique individual, with a mind, body, and spirit that are intertwined. We all have the power to heal ourselves. It is my belief and hope that the information in this book will help you direct that power, enabling you to live a longer life, brimming with natural health, energy, and happiness.

AYURVEDA

A WORD ABOUT THE LANGUAGE

The original Ayurvedic texts were written in Sanskrit, the language of ancient India. (It is now used only for sacred or scholarly writings.) Many of the original Sanskrit terms have survived the translation into English and are used by practitioners in talking and writing about Ayurveda. We have kept the use of Sanskrit words to a minimum to avoid confusion. However, it is impossible to avoid Sanskrit words completely, because sometimes there is simply no adequate translation into English, or the translation is awkward. One example is the word dosha, which means literally "that which has a fault" and is often translated as "governing principle." Other examples are the names of the three types of doshas, vata, pitta, and kapha—these have no translation at all. Another is prakruti, which some writers and practitioners translate as "constitution," or "body type," or "personality," or "biotype," or even "psychophysiological constitution." Some of these terms are a mouthful without being quite accurate. In these and a handful of other instances we prefer to give a thorough explanation of the concept when it is first introduced and then use the much more beautiful, precise, and poetic Sanskrit term thereafter. You will soon feel comfortable referring to the doshas and your prakruti, much as everyone now talks familiarly of cholesterol and aerobic exercise, terms that took some getting used to when they were first introduced.

PART ONE

UNDERSTANDING AYURVEDA

8

AYURVEDA

CHAPTER ONE

THE BACKGROUND AND PHILOSOPHY OF AYURVEDA

Ayurveda, the oldest known disease-prevention and health care system, is the original holistic medicine. It is based on a view of the world and of life that draws directly on nature. According to this view, the elements, forces, and principles that comprise all of nature —and that hold it together and make it function—are also seen in human beings. In Ayurveda the mind (or consciousness) and the body (or physical matter) not only influence each other—they are each other. Together they form the mind-body. The universal consciousness is an intelligent, aware ocean of energy that gives rise to the physical world we perceive through our five senses. Ayurvedic philosophy and practices connect us to every aspect of ourselves and remind us that we are connected to every aspect of nature, each other, and the entire universe.

There can be no mental health without physical health, and vice versa. It should come as no surprise, then, that in Ayurveda, symptoms and diseases that could be categorized as mental thoughts or feelings are just as important as symptoms and diseases of the physical body. Both are due to imbalances within a person, and both are treated by restoring the natural balance—mentally and physically—that is our birthright. In Ayurveda your whole life and lifestyle must be in harmony before you can enjoy true well being.

Ayurveda is a Sanskrit word that literally translated means "science of life" or "practices of longevity." It emphasizes prevention of disease, rejuvenation of our body systems, and extension of life span. The profound premise and promise of Ayurveda is that through certain practices not only can we prevent heart disease and make our headaches go away, but we can also better understand ourselves and the world around us, live a long healthy life in balance and harmony, achieve our fullest potential, and express our true inner nature on a daily basis.

Of course if you are taking medication or are under medical care for a diagnosed condition, you should consult your physician before taking any Ayurvedic remedies. Serious illnesses caused by severe imbalances are best treated by a professional. However, the foundation of Ayurveda is self-knowledge and self-healing. Thus it is supremely suited for self-care of minor imbalances and ailments and as an adjunct to professional medical care. It is compatible with conventional medicine and with other forms of natural medicine, such as homeopathy, and includes health-building practices such as exercise, massage, meditation, and nutrition as well as gentle herbal remedies. Imagine greeting every day with a soothing massage, eating fresh, seasonal, deliciously spiced foods, and regularly taking time out to close your eyes, relax, and get in touch with your deepest self. As you will see, Ayurveda is a system of pleasures, not deprivations.

THE A-Z GUIDE

A "NEW" OLD VIEW OF HEALTH AND DISEASE

Until recently modern Western medicine believed that health was simply the absence of disease. Illness was caused purely by something outside the body, the way a hammer hitting your toe causes pain—viruses caused colds, allergens caused allergies, stress caused anxiety, carcinogens caused cancer, and so on. The solution was to find the right pill and the disease would be cured.

But today we know that the seeds of illness are sown way before obvious symptoms appear. The absence of a readily diagnosable disease is no longer the definition of health—people want to feel good, not just "not bad." The hammer-hitting-the-toe model of disease doesn't explain the wide variation in people's abilities to resist illness or recover from illness. When you encounter a cold virus, you have only one chance in eight of getting a cold. Seven out of eight times your mind-body is able to defend itself. Clearly the virus is only one small factor—the state of your general health is paramount.

By focusing on physical cause and effect Western medicine has looked at individual organs in isolation, as separate from one another and from the mind and spirit. By way of contrast ancient civilizations were intimately in touch with their nonphysical selves and had rich inner lives. They knew what modern science is just now starting to realize: The mind and body are so connected as to be indistinguishable from each other.

In many ways modern science is only beginning to catch up with Ayurveda. For example research is discovering that certain people are constitutionally predisposed to certain illnesses, and proving that lifestyle practices and gentle herbal medicines can make a huge difference in our ability to resist disease, recover from illness, and extend our lives. That's exactly what the ancient science of Ayurveda has been saying for thousands of years.

Many studies show that meditation, a cornerstone practice in Ayurveda, has a wide variety of effects on the body. A 1996 study, published by the

AYURVEDA

American Heart Association, showed that meditation significantly reduced high blood pressure, a major risk factor in heart disease and stroke. Another study, of two thousand meditators, conducted in 1987 found that meditators visited doctors half as often as the average nonmeditating American and had lower-than-normal rates for cancer and heart attacks.

Although the Ayurvedic worldview includes a religious component, in this book we are not concerned with the religious philosophy. You can meditate, do yoga, take herbs, and incorporate the five-sense therapies into your life without accepting the particular spiritual tenets of ancient India. As Dr. David Frawley, a world-renowned Vedic teacher, writes in his book Ayurvedic Healing, "What we do every day is our real religion, for it shows what we value in life."

SIX THOUSAND YEARS OF HEALTH AND HEALING

Ayurveda has its roots in the ancient civilization of the Indian city states that flourished six thousand years ago. This vast, prosperous civilization spread over 500,000 square miles (larger than England, France, and Germany combined), and developed sophisticated systems of pictograph communications, weights and measures, and refined governmental organizations. Two of the largest cities had populations ranging from twenty thousand to fifty thousand. The cities were laid out in square blocks larger than those in New York City, with rows of brick houses and drainage and sewage systems far advanced for their time.

Ayurveda was the system of health care conceived and developed by the seers (risbie) and natural scientists through centuries of observations, experiments, discussions, and meditations. For several thousand years their teachings were passed on orally from teacher to student; about the fifth to sixth century B.C., elaborately detailed texts were written in Sanskrit, the ancient language of India. For many years Ayurveda flourished and was used by rich and poor alike in India and Southeast Asia.

However in A.D. 1200 Muslims conquered the area and added their influence to Ayurveda. In the 1800s the British colonized India and discouraged Ayurveda by shutting down Ayurvedic hospitals. By the mid 1900s city dwellers had been converted to Western medicine, and Ayurveda was considered a folk medicine used mostly by the rural population.

But Ayurveda is now enjoying a comeback. Many books on the subject were written in the 1960s, and books are still being written today—a further testament to the resiliency and power of Ayurveda. In India more than one hundred colleges are graduating an increasing number of Ayurvedic physicians. And the state is conducting research into natural treatments for chronic disease.

THE AYURVEDIC VIEW OF HEALTH AND DISEASE

Like Western science and the health philosophies of many other cultures, Ayurveda is part of a larger attempt to understand and explain the world and how all the parts in it function. Why does the sun rise? How do plants and animals grow? Why do some people live to a ripe old age while others die young? Why do some people get cancer and others heart disease? Why does your uncle Joe devour green peppers when this food doesn't at all agree with you? Why are some people rich and others poor? Why do some forms of music excite or agitate you and others instill a calm peacefulness?

Ayurveda, like all philosophies, is a worldview or model that tries to make order and sense out of life. It may seem a bit confusing initially. The Sanskrit terms may sound unfamiliar, but they are necessary because

AYURVEDA

Ayurveda represents a new way of looking at life. Modern Western thinking is basically linear: A causes B to happen, which in turn causes C and so on, in a step-like straight line. Ayurvedic thinking is circular in that everything affects everything else and concepts flow back and forth without end. The in-depth study and practice of Ayurveda is a lifelong endeavor. However, the basic principles of Ayurveda are easy to grasp because they are simple and you can observe them directly in your daily life.

As you learn about this system, more and more of the principles will fall into place. With the clarity and deepening understanding that comes with everyday practice, you become a seer, a seeker of truth, a scientist, using yourself and the world as your laboratory in which to test the veracity of its principles. Learn about Ayurveda, integrate the practices into your life—and observe. Does Ayurveda help you get to know yourself better? Does it help you make better sense of the world, your feelings, your health, your behavior? Do you feel better mentally and physically? This is the true test of whether any particular approach to health and healing works or not.

Your journey begins with an understanding of the three doshas, the fundamental forces that form the basis for all prevention, diagnosis, and treatment of illness in Ayurveda.

THE THREE DOSHAS (GOVERNING PRINCIPLES)

Ayurveda recognizes five basic elements, or constituents, to be the smallest components to which anything can be reduced. They are air, space, fire, water, and earth. Everything in nature is composed of these five glorious, mysterious, essential components—including humans.

AIR is the Ayurvedic term for the gaseous form of matter.

THE A-Z GUIDE

SPACE (sometimes called ether) is the expanse or area in which air is contained and through which it moves.

FIRE is the radiant form of matter and is needed for any process of transformation, or "digestion."

WATER is used to describe the liquid form of matter.

EARTH is the solid form of matter and is responsible for groundedness and solidity.

The five elements, in infinite combinations and proportions, are the basis of all life-forms and things, with three forces to keep the elements in the right relationship with one another. The three forces, the doshas, govern all the functions of the body, mind, and universal consciousness.

The three doshas, or governing principles, are called vata, pitta, and kapha. Each dosha has its own set of characteristics, which arise out of the elements from which they are made. This includes the physical and emotional characteristics and personality traits of people, as well as of everything else. For example there are vata, pitta, and kapha kinds of flowers, people, houses, music, foods, trees, birds, and bees, as well as times of day and seasons.

Every person (and thing) contains all three doshas. However, the proportion varies according to the individual, and usually one or two doshas predominate. Within each person the doshas are continually interacting with one another and with the doshas in all of nature. This interplay among the fundamental forces and components explains why people can have much in common but also have an endless variety of individual differences in the way they behave and respond to their environment. Ayurveda recognizes that different foods, tastes, colors, and sounds affect the doshas in different ways. For example very hot and pungent spices aggravate pitta; but cold, light foods such as salads calm it down. This ability to affect the doshas is the underlying basis for Ayurvedic practices and therapies.

AYURVEDA

The doshas are abstract ideas, invisible themselves but evident everywhere you look once you are aware of them. Physicists can't fully explain the phenomena known as gravity and magnetism, yet we can see and feel their power to pull and push things around. So it is with vata, pitta, and kapha. As you become more familiar with the qualities of each dosha, you'll be able to see them at work in yourself, your family and friends, animals, the weather, and even food and technology. You will learn more about the doshas throughout this book. Here are brief introductory descriptions:

VATA is composed of the elements air and space; air, the dominant element, is contained within the spaces and channels of the body. Vata governs your physical and psychological movement, flow, circulation, and activities of the nervous system. People who are predominantly vata resemble air and space (or wind as it is sometimes referred to). They tend to be thin, quick, light, changeable, unpredictable, enthusiastic, and talkative. When they are out of balance, they experience diseases of the nervous system; scattered energy; intestinal gas and constipation; insomnia; dry, flaky skin; and anxiety. Vata governs the life force within us and thus leads the other two doshas.

PITTA is composed of fire and water; fire, the main element, is contained within the protective waters of the body (such as digestive enzymes). It governs your metabolism—body processes involving heat, digestion, and hormones, and biochemical reactions such as those required to produce energy. When pitta predominates, a person tends to be fiery: intense, with a sharp and creative mind, a penetrating look in their eyes, a reddish or easily flushed complexion, a competitive streak, and a hot temper. Their illnesses are related to inflammation, such as heartburn, ulcers, skin rashes, anger, and irritation.

KAPHA is composed of earth and water; water, the main element, is contained within the body's mass, or earth. It governs your body's structure and tissues and maintains stability, cohesion, fluid balance, and biological strength. Kapha types are solid and steady, even-tempered and calm, with impressive endurance and a large body size that tends to gain

THE A-Z GUIDE

weight. Imbalances in kapha predispose you to diseases of the respiratory system, sinus problems, obesity, tumors, mental and physical lethargy, and a tendency to procrastinate.

The idea that there are certain body types has also appeared in Western thinking. For example in the area of weight control and body shape, people have been categorized as endomorphs (soft and rounded), mesomorphs (muscular and bony), and ectomorphs (lean and sinewy). And the notion that individuals have differing innate vulnerabilities to certain diseases has also gained a foothold in modern medicine. Some may be determined by inherited genetic makeup, which may also be linked with more discernible characteristics or markers. The notion of the hard-driving, perfectionist type-A personality who gets ulcers and heart attacks is one example. Scientists have also noticed that people who accumulate weight around the waist are more prone to heart attack than those who gain weight around the hips. However, the concept of the doshas and their relation to health is much more holistic, integrated, subtle, and complex than any of these ideas.

MAINTAINING BALANCE ALONG THE DYNAMIC JOURNEY OF LIFE

Your individual constitution—the unique proportion of the three doshas that you were born with—is called your prakruti. Your prakruti is your true, essential nature. No dosha is inherently better than any other, and no proportion of doshas is more desirable than any other. We need them all and we need them to be in balance, as determined by your prakruti, in order to function and sustain health.

But life is not static. As the saying goes, "Stuff happens." Your doshas are always fluctuating by interacting with other doshas in the world—stress, food, pollution, the noise or view outside your window, changes in the season, and other factors. As a result health is a dynamic process of continually making small adjustments to compensate.

AYURVEDA

You can experience this dynamism when you do balancing yoga poses, in which you can feel your physical body undergo subtle changes to maintain equilibrium; and during meditation, in which your mind continually returns its attention to your mantra as thoughts and feelings draw it away.

Your current condition is called your vikruti. Although it reflects your ability to adjust to life's influences and is always changing, it should match your prakruti, or inborn constitution, as closely as possible. If the current proportion of your doshas differs significantly from your constitutional proportion, it indicates imbalances, which in turn can lead to illness.

Think of your prakruti as the immutable road you were placed on at birth. Then think of your vikruti as the dynamic life journey you are taking on that road. In my clinic we find that often the first step toward vibrant health is to understand your essence, to accept yourself for who you are, and then to follow the path that best supports your true nature. Although your road is not so narrow as to be rigid, it represents the best path that you, as a unique individual, need to follow. It is nature providing you with your own guideline to well-being. Stray too far off the road and that way lies ill health—you may be more vulnerable to digestive problems, respiratory infections, cancer, heart disease, or depression. But if you stay on the road, you'll encounter smoother traveling and better health.

In the next chapter we provide you with self-assessments—tests to help you determine your prakruti and your vikruti. The Ayurvedic practices and lifestyle patterns provided in subsequent chapters are designed to gently lead your mind-body back to the road that's best for you. Although in making these life changes you will notice some improvement right away, others will take longer. Ayurveda acknowledges that illness doesn't happen overnight. It takes years of accumulated imbalances and mini-breakdowns brought on by poor digestion, stress, and other lifestyle habits.

THE A-Z GUIDE

"DIGESTING" FOOD AND ALL OF LIFE

According to Ayurveda, digestion is the cornerstone of health because good digestion nourishes the body. Eating the proper foods will make a big difference in your well-being. However, in Ayurveda we are concerned not only with the material food you ingest, digest, and assimilate, nor only with the organs of your digestive system. The impact of what you see, hear, taste, smell, feel, and think is also important. In a sense all you experience and take into your mind-body needs to be "well digested" and distributed to all the cells of the body. Remember, everything in your environment is composed of doshas that interact with your own doshas.

Agni: Your Digestive Fire

One of the most fundamental concepts in Ayurveda is that of agni. Agni is the digestive and metabolic "fire" produced by the doshas that grabs the essence of nourishment from food, feelings, and thoughts and transforms it into a form your body can use. Through the heat of agni, various tissues of the body produce secretions, metabolic reactions, and other processes needed to create energy and maintain and repair the body. Agni is also part of the immune system since its heat destroys harmful organisms and toxins. The activity of agni varies throughout the day and, as you'll learn in later chapters, maintaining the strength and natural ebb and flow of your digestive fires is needed for good digestion, good immune function, and resistance to disease. Agni is needed to form ojas.

Ojas: The Substance That Maintains Life

Ojas is the by-product of a healthy, efficient, contented physiology. It is the "juice" that remains after food has been properly digested and assimilated. When you are producing ojas, it means all your organs have integrated vitality and you are receiving the nourishment your mind and body need. Your whole being hums with good vibrations because you are producing and feeling bliss, not pain. However, when your agni isn't working properly, you don't produce ojas. Instead food, thoughts, and feelings turn into ama.

Ama: Toxins

Ama arises from improperly digested toxic particles that clog the channels in your body. Some of these channels are physical and include the intestines, lymphatic system, arteries and veins, capillaries, and genitourinary tract. Others are nonphysical channels called nadis through which your energy flows. Ama toxicity accumulates wherever there is a weakness in the body, and this will allow a genetic predisposition to overtake you and create disease or keep it going. While Ayurveda offers ways you can cleanse the body of ama, it's best to prevent it from forming in the first place. You know you've got an ama problem if your tongue is coated or if you are feeling tired all the time.

Malas: Waste Products

Malas are the waste products of your body and include urine, feces, mucus, and sweat. Eliminating waste is crucial to good health, but dosha imbalances stifle the flow of the malas, creating a toxic internal environment. If you are not eliminating malas, it means you are accumulating ama somewhere in your system.

Prana: The Life Force

Another key concept in Ayurveda is the life force that enters the body at birth and travels through all the parts of the body until it leaves at the moment of death.

STRESS AND DISEASE

In order to fully appreciate the powerful role of Ayurveda in restoring health, you need to understand how it helps you handle stress, which is at

THE A-Z GUIDE

the root of many ailments big and small. Dr. Hans Selye, the pioneering researcher who practically invented the concept of stress, defined it rather poetically: "Stress is anything from a passionate embrace to a boring game of chess." Of course it is also a sock to the jaw, a pink slip, a divorce, a ring in your teenage daughter's nose (or your own parents' not letting you have a nose ring). Stress can be a windowless office with an uncomfortable chair or the knowledge that our species is destroying the natural environment.

Stress, then, can be anything that comes knocking on your door, but it is not necessarily the Big Bad Wolf himself, threatening to blow your house down. Rather the Big Bad Wolf is within you; it is your reaction to any event you believe to be stressful. You can either digest the stressful feelings and convert them to useful energy that helps you grow and develop or you can have trouble digesting stress and create ama, which tires out and depletes the nervous system and overworks the immune system, which in turn leaves the door open to illness.

So what happens when we are under stress? When we perceive something to be stressful, an internal alarm goes off, triggering a cascade of physiological changes that was originally described by Selye as a fight-or-flight response. Adrenaline floods the bloodstream, the heart beats faster; digestion screeches to a halt, muscles tense up, blood pressure skyrockets, the brain and senses become hyper alert. This response is designed to enable to us to fight for our lives or to get us away from the danger as fast as possible. It worked well for our ancestors because their stressors were mainly of the saber-toothed-tiger variety. Stresses were immediate and short-lived, and once the dangerous situation was over, the body was designed to return to normal.

Today life is not so simple or clear-cut. Instead a saber-toothed tigers we're continually barraged by little day-to-day hassles—job insecurity or frustration, exasperating children, traffic jams, lack of fulfillment—that are difficult to fight or escape from. Nor is the stress response so simple and clear-cut. We now know that the way a person responds to stressful situations depends in part on the way he or she has learned to cope. Even

AYURVEDA

the so-called negative emotions depicted in the topmost section of the Lion pose illustration aren't necessarily harmful. Fear, anger, and so on—these are all good, natural human emotions under certain conditions. But if they are not resolved and metabolized by your agni (that is, "digested"), they become stressful. The more stress we perceive, and the less able we are to cope with it, the less we are able to recover from it, and the less we are able to deal with new stressors.

Prolonged stress wreaks all sorts of havoc: It can contribute to fatigue, diabetes, hypertension, ulcers, loss of libido, and reduced resistance to disease. Emotional upset can throw women's periods off kilter, reduce fertility, and make menopause more difficult. Feeling stressed affects your ability to work, to think clearly, and to have satisfying social relationships. In animal experiments stress has accelerated aging and death, hastened the spread of cancer, and promoted heart attacks. In 1993 the U.S. Public Health Survey estimated that 70 to 80 percent of Americans who visit physicians suffer from a stress-related disorder.

That the thoughts in your mind have an enormous effect on your body has become well accepted. There's even a tongue-twisting name for a new field of scientific investigation of the mind-body connection: psychoneuroimmunology or PNI. PNI studies the interaction between the mind, nervous system, immune system, and endocrine system and acknowledges the unity of our complex interacting parts.

Early mind-body studies showed that people were more likely to become ill after suffering severe emotional trauma; recent studies have been able to actually measure the dip in immune defenses. In one study the immune cells of students dropped significantly during exam week, presumably because of the extra stress. In another, rats were taught to shut down their own immune systems by conditioning alone. In 1990 a Stanford University Medical Center psychiatrist who set out to disprove the mind-body link provided strong evidence that it does exist. In the study, women with advanced breast cancer attended support groups in which they shared feelings and information and learned simple relaxation techniques. When compared with women who did not attend the groups, the supported women were less depressed, felt less pain, had a more positive outlook—and lived twice as long. Two of the women were still alive and disease-free ten years later, but none of the unsupported women survived. Many scientists suspect that the mind-body connection is involved in the documented spontaneous remissions from cancer and many other diseases that appear to be otherwise inexplicable.

As a result of these and other experiments, modern immunobiologists routinely refer to the immune system as a circulating nervous system. Needless to say, this has immense significance in our daily lives. Press your fingertips to your lymph glands. Do they feel hard and tender? If so, your nervous system is communicating to you that it is tired. One system is expressing the state of another, seemingly separate system.

In Ayurveda restoring and revitalizing the stress-prone nervous system is the key to preventing and treating all disease. This approach offers tools and technology to reach the underlying sources of illness—stress in its many forms: from bacteria, viruses, and parasites to toxic pollution and toxic emotions.

AYURVEDA

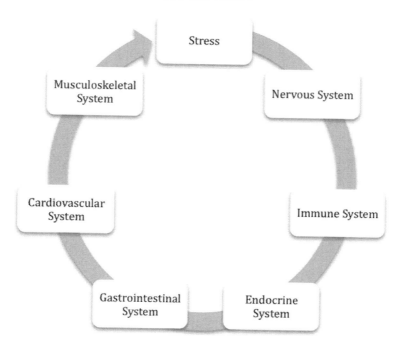

The mind-body is a never-ending cycle of feelings, nerve impulses, hormonal secretions, and biochemical reactions. Your systems are constantly interacting not only with the world, but with themselves and one another. Unresolved stress (whether blissful or painful) leaves the "fight-or-flight" response stuck in the "ON" position. This wear and tear exhausts first the nervous system, then the endocrine system and the immune system, and eventually affects all the other systems, leaving you vulnerable to infection and other diseases.

As a result it can help with minor annoying everyday ailments as well as serious conditions, as attested to by the following patient:

> "After suffering for over forty years with asthma, allergies, pain, and chronic fatigue due to years of taking antibiotics, Ayurveda has given me a quality of life I had never before experienced."

Although you may be tempted to let your practice slide during times of acute stress, those are the very times you need the calming, balancing practices of Ayurveda, as another patient discovered:

THE A-Z GUIDE

"Recently my father had a heart attack. I was able to keep my anxiety and fears under control by practicing all the vata-balancing techniques Dr. Thomas taught me. Instead of falling apart and becoming a hindrance, I was able to nurture myself both physically and emotionally and be there when my father needed me so desperately."

CONSIDER THE POSSIBILITIES

The goal of Ayurveda is to get in touch with the interactions of your doshas, with other people, and with the rhythms of the universe. When you bring your mind and awareness to that, and feel the universe flowing through you twenty-four hours a day, you are experiencing wholeness. This is why, as Deepak Chopra points out, there is no wear and tear in the universe—only rest, activity, and endless cycles of renewal and transformation.

As you read this, your mind-body is busily renewing itself. You know from experience that you constantly need to cut your hair and clip your nails. As Dr. Deepak Chopra points out, what you may not know is that . . .

- Ninety-eight percent of the atoms in your body are replaced each year.
- The bones in your skeleton regenerate every three months.
- The cells of your liver are made new every six weeks.
- You generate a whole new skin once a month.
- Your stomach lining is replaced every five days.

What this indicates is that if you feed yourself with the right "foods," you can influence the regeneration process. In the computer world there is a saying, "Garbage in, garbage out." It's the same with your mind-body. Instead of a limp, tired undernourished turnover of cells, you can enjoy a strong, vital one. Ayurvedic practices guide you toward supplying your

AYURVEDA

mind-body with diverse, pure, high-octane fuel and burning it cleanly, which leads to an improved healing process and a return to health.

Our relationship to the elements, the doshas, and the senses connects us to endless cycles of transformation within. This is the wisdom, the paradigm, of Ayurveda. It can become a part of your daily life.

CHAPTER TWO
GETTING TO KNOW YOUR DOSHAS

As you learned in the previous chapter, the five elements combine to form the three principal forces, the doshas. Each person contains all three doshas, which must be kept in balance for that person to remain healthy. The ideal state for you to be in is your prakruti, your essential nature, which consists of the proportions of the doshas that nature gave you when you were born.

However, the health of the body is not like a clock; it is not a perfectly predictable mechanism. It is a dynamic, moving, interactive flux, and your vikruti is a reflection of this process. Your vikruti is your current condition, and when this differs significantly from your prakruti, you experience symptoms—signs that something is awry in your mind-body. Determining your prakruti and vikruti puts you in touch with both your unchanging essence (prakruti) and the patterns, cycles, and tendencies in your changeable nature (vikruti) that can lead to imbalances, symptoms, and serious disease. You can then use this information to follow the general Ayurvedic practices as well as specific remedies to coax your doshas back to whatever proportion is normal for you. Once you are back in balance, you can embark on the lifetime maintenance regimen designed to keep your prakruti in balance.

SELF-ASSESSMENT: YOUR DOSHAS, YOUR SELF

In this chapter we provide self-assessment tests to help you determine first your vikruti and then your prakruti. They contain the same types of questions an Ayurvedic physician would ask you during a consultation. In both assessments we start with the symptoms and characteristics of the mind, emotions, and behavior; this is in order to counteract the tendency that most people have to concentrate almost exclusively on the state of their bodies. We want to shift the emphasis so that the immaterial aspects of health get at least as much attention as the physical ones. We also hope that getting you to think about your mind, emotions, and behavior will put you in a frame of mind that allows a more open, freer mode of evaluation. In this mode it's more likely you will be more objective about your physical attributes, rather than base your answers on your likes and dislikes about your body and how you would prefer it to be.

Taking the Tests

Self-assessment and self-knowledge is a key concept in Ayurveda and is what attracts many people to this system in the first place. But at this point you may wonder: Do I really have to take all these tests to get rid of my headache, insomnia, or digestive problems? Can't I just take the Ayurvedic remedies right now? It is possible to get relief from these symptoms and the others listed in the A–Z section simply by following our suggestions for the herbal and five-sense remedies. In fact using specific remedies lets you get your feet wet and is the way many people discover how effective Ayurveda can be. However, while these specific, gentle Ayurvedic remedies are an improvement over commonly used drugs that are sold with or without prescription, which can be harsh or ineffective, they are a limited form of Ayurveda.

We urge you to go beyond this simple use of Ayurveda in order to reap long-term as well as immediate rewards. Not only will the specific remedies work much more effectively to relieve your symptoms, but you will enjoy the additional benefits of Ayurveda: self-knowledge, disease prevention, rejuvenation, and longevity.

Going beyond symptom-specific remedies means integrating fundamental Ayurvedic practices into your life on a daily basis. That is why under each A–Z entry we also recommend that you follow the Daily Lifestyle Regimen (see Chapter 6) designed to generally balance your predominant dosha. These regimens individualize the Ayurvedic practices and techniques described in chapters 3 and 4—including recommendations for food and herbal teas, meditation, yoga, and exercise—by tailoring them to each dosha. These fundamental practices strengthen your underlying constitution and treat the whole person and your overall disease pattern, not just the symptom. In order to get the most out of these techniques, then, you need to know your doshas and how they express themselves within your prakruti and vikruti.

There are other advantages to determining your prakruti and vikruti as well. Understanding who you are, why you are the way you are, and how outside influences affect you physically and emotionally familiarizes you with the positive and negative characteristics of your doshas. Such understanding is wonderfully liberating—instead of judging yourself and others, of wanting to change or "break" yourself or other people, you can develop a love and tolerance as well as a whole set of tools that allows you to encourage the positive aspects of your doshas to emerge. You can better recognize the negative characteristics in the future and take appropriate steps to balance them on a daily basis, before symptoms set in. And you have a consistent means of measuring positive changes. A patient of mine says,

> "Ayurveda is transforming my life. It is helping me to become a healthier, happier person who knows and understands herself, others, and her environment on a deeper, more compassionate level than ever before."

To begin, take each test on its own sheet of paper, allowing one column for each dosha. Use the Record Sheet provided to enter your scores and keep track of your progress. It's also a good idea to date and identify each worksheet with the appropriate heading such as "Vikruti: Mind-Emotions-Behavior" and save them so that you can refer to them (as well as your Record Sheet) and see more precisely where the improvement is occurring.

SIX STEPS TO BALANCED DOSHAS

Here's a summary of the process, which is explained in greater detail later in the chapter:

STEP 1. Determine Your Vikruti

Using the self-assessments, determine your initial vikruti so that you know where you stand now.

STEP 2. Determine Your Prakruti

Using the self-assessments, determine your prakruti so that you know what you are aiming for.

STEP 3. Determine the Imbalance

Following two simple rules of thumb, determine where your major imbalance is.

THE A-Z GUIDE

STEP 4. Stabilize Your Doshas

Use general Ayurvedic practices to establish a Daily Lifestyle Regimen to stabilize the dosha that is your major source of imbalance. In addition use specific Ayurvedic herbal remedies and five-sense remedies for alleviating key symptoms.

STEP 5. Monitor Your Progress

Follow these general and specific practices until the symptoms subside, monitoring your improvement by repeating the vikruti test every three months.

STEP 6. Maintain Balance

When your symptoms have subsided and the ratio of the doshas in your vikruti have come close to those in your prakruti, you need only follow the appropriate Daily Lifestyle Regimen. If old symptoms return, or new ones appear, use the specific remedies recommended for those conditions in the A-Z section.

Examples of how this works for real-life people are included at the end of the chapter.

What Do We Mean by "Balancing" the Doshas?

Many practitioners and books on Ayurveda talk about balancing the doshas. This term is somewhat confusing, because it could be interpreted as trying to give yourself equal amounts of all three. Not only is that impossible—it would be going against your inborn nature—but it would be quite dull to have everyone so similar! The idea is to find the "balance" that is right for you, first by correcting any severe imbalances in your vikruti and then by maintaining your new balanced condition by following the daily routine that's tailored to your prakruti. Another term

AYURVEDA

used frequently is pacifying the doshas. This, too, is not quite accurate because a dosha could be depleted rather than aggravated, in which case you want to elevate it, not calm it down. That's why we prefer to use the term stabilize—this more accurately reflects what Ayurvedic practices are really trying to do. By stabilizing aggravated or diminished doshas, you create the balance you seek.

STEP 1: DETERMINE YOUR CURRENT CONDITION (VIKRUTI)

This will answer the question, "What's out of balance that needs stabilizing?" Take this part of the test once now and then again every three months to monitor your progress. When determining your vikruti, identify your problem areas by focusing on symptoms that are occurring now or that have occurred consistently within the last" two weeks. The lists we have provided are not all the possible symptoms you might experience; rather they represent those most typical of the particular doshas because this is the best way to target imbalances. There are many more symptoms that are common to all three doshas—for example, headache—but that have subtly different characteristics.

Note that the symptoms in the test reflect the elements that comprise the doshas. For example, vata imbalances reflect the drying, airy, disruptive powers of the wind. Pitta imbalances reflect the burning action of fire. Kapha imbalances reflect the heaviness and stagnation of water. The location of the symptoms are also clues. Although all three doshas are found in every cell in every part of the body, doshas tend to concentrate in certain areas, and therefore symptoms tend to occur in those parts of the body where the dosha dwells. Vata is primarily found in the lower part of the torso, particularly in the colon; intestinal gas, pain, or constipation is a telltale sign of a vata imbalance. Pitta is primarily found in the middle third of the torso, and the small intestine is considered to be the seat; imbalances show up as burning sensations (heartburn, ulcers) in the digestive tract. Kapha, on the other hand, dwells mostly in the

THE A-Z GUIDE

upper part of the torso, and thus aggravated kapha often produces chest problems such as congestion. However, this is not an iron clad rule, since the doshas permeate the body and their interaction can push and pull symptoms to distant sites.

Scoring

As you take the test, score yourself based on how often the symptom has occurred in the last week or two, and whether the symptom is strong, moderate, or weak. Use the following scale:

3 = Strong, frequent
2 = Moderate
1= Weak, infrequent
0 = Not at all

AYURVEDA

VIKRUTI: MENTAL-EMOTIONAL-BEHAVIORAL SYMPTOMS

IS YOUR VATA AGGRAVATED?	IS YOUR PITTA AGGRAVATED?	IS YOUR KAPHA AGGRAVATED?
Worried	Angry	Sluggish thinking
Tired, yet wired	Irritable	Dull thinking
Can't relax	Hostile	Groggy all day
Can't concentrate	Enraged	Apathetic, no desire
Anxious, fearful	Destructive Impatient	Depressed
Nervous	Critical of self and others	Slow to comprehend
Agitated mind		Sad
Impatient	Argumentative	Slow to react
Spaced-out Self-defeating	Bossy, controlling	Procrastinating
	Frustrated	Clingy, hanging on to people and ideas
Antsy or hyperactive	Willful	
Shy, insecure	Aggressive	Sentimental Greedy
Restless	Vain	Possessive
Indecisive	Reckless	Materialistic

THE A-Z GUIDE

VIKRUTI: PHYSICAL SYMPTOMS AND ILLNESSES

IS YOUR VATA AGGRAVATED?	IS YOUR PITTA AGGRAVATED?	IS YOUR KAPHA AGGRAVATED?
Weight loss, underweight	Acid stomach, heartburn	Lethargy
Fatigue, poor stamina	Stomach ulcer	Sleeping too much
Insomnia, wake up at night and can't go back to sleep	Fitful sleep	Very tired in the morning, hard to get out of bed
Generalized aches, sharp pains	Diarrhea	Drowsy or groggy during the day
Agitated movement	Bad breath	Weight gain, obesity
Very sensitive to cold	Very sensitive to heat	Mucus and congestion in the chest or throat
Nail biting	Hot flashes	Mucus and congestion in the nose or sinuses
Rough, flaky skin	Skin rashes	Nausea
Chapped lips	Boils"	Diabetes
Fainting spells	Bloodshot eyes Acne	Hay fever
Heart palpitations	Sour body odor	Pale, cool, clammy skin
Arthritis, stiff and painful joints	Disturbing dreams	Edema, water retention
Constipation	Night sweats	Bloated feeling
Intestinal bloating, gas	Weakness due to low blood sugar	Sluggish digestion, food "just sits" in the stomach
Belching, hiccups	Food allergies	High cholesterol
Dry, sore throat	Fevers	Aching joints
Dry eyes		

AYURVEDA

STEP 2: DETERMINE YOUR MIND-BODY CONSTITUTION (PRAKRUTI)

The prakruti is a guideline to your natural state and your potential. This test will answer the question, what's your essential nature? To get the most accurate determination, do the entire self-assessment once, now. Then retest yourself two more times, once every three days. Add up the totals within each dosha and divide by three to get the average. Your emotions—and your perception of them—tend to fluctuate more than your physical characteristics do, and this multiple testing will give you a truer picture. In Ayurveda a physician would take your pulse three times before determining your prakruti; so in testing yourself three times, you are being a good physician.

Because the vikruti often throws the prakruti out of balance, it may be difficult for you to get in touch with your true essence. You may need to go back and think about how you were when you were younger, sometimes as far back as your childhood. You may want to ask friends and relatives for their impressions of you then and now. (This will be quite interesting all by itself—many people are astonished to hear how another person sees them, when compared with their own self-view.) Even then it may be difficult to get an accurate picture because some people are influenced early on to suppress parts of themselves. For example a young child with a pitta prakruti may have been taught to suppress her temper tantrums and instead be "good" to get what she wants. So instead of crying, kicking, and turning red with anger, she experiences angry red skin rashes and inflammations all her life and also suffers vata symptoms from the stress of suppressing her true nature. (See "Ayurveda and Your Child," which teaches parents how to avoid suppressing their children's true nature.)

THE A-Z GUIDE

Scoring

When scoring, use the following scale

3 = Frequently, severe
2 = Sometimes, moderate 1= Rarely, mild
0 = Never or almost never

The dosha with the highest number is the predominant dosha in your prakruti.

PRAKRUTI: MIND-EMOTIONS-BEHAVIOR

	VATA	PITTA	KAPHA
I am	Flexible, optimistic, lively, intuitive, enthusiastic, changeable, an initiator	Ambitious, practical, intense, motivated, perceptive, warm, friendly, independent, courageous, discriminating, a good leader, goal-oriented, competitive	Calm, peaceful, solicitous, resilient, content, loyal, slow, deliberate, relaxed, compassionate, patient, nurturing, stable
My memory is	Quick to remember—and to forget	Average, clear, distinct	Slow to Remember and to forget

AYURVEDA

	VATA	**PITTA**	**KAPHA**
My thinking style is	Restless, quick	Organized, efficient, accurate	Slow, methodical, exacting
I process information	Quickly	At medium speed	Slowly
My creativity level is	Filled with ideas, but tends to follow through poorly	Inventive in many areas, with good follow-through	Best in the field of business
Under stress I become	Anxious, insecure, tense, and sigh and hyperventilate	Aggressive, angry, irritable, headachy, nauseated	Lethargic, dull, in denial
I dream of	Activity, running, flying, frightening things	Violence, fire, anger, passion, the sun	Romance, sentimentality, water and snow
My speech pattern is	Fast, talkative	Precise, convincing	Slow, monotones, melodic
My voice sounds	Weak, low, hoarse, whiny	Sharp, loud, high-pitched, penetrating	Pleasant, deep, resonant
My lifestyle is	Highly active	Active	Rather inactive

THE A-Z GUIDE

	VATA	PITTA	KAPHA
My spending habits are	Wasteful, can't save, throw money away on trifles	Moderate, can save, but spend money on luxuries	Thrifty, accumulate wealth but spend money on food
My sex drive is	Either in very high or very low gear	Moderate frequency, but passionate and domineering	Infrequent, constant or cyclic, loyal and devoted
I dislike weather that is	Cold, windy, dry	Hot, with strong sun	Cool and damp
When making decisions I am	Unsure	Quick and decisive	Deliberate
Emotionally, I	Worry, am anxious, moody, and emotional	Get angry and irritated easily	Stay calm, complacent, get angry slowly
I love	Traveling, art, esoteric subjects	Sports, politics, luxury	Good food
The pace of my activity is	Fast	Medium speed, intense	Slow, steady

AYURVEDA

PRAKRUTI: BODY CHARACTERISTICS

	VATA	PITTA	KAPHA
My bone structure is	Slim, slight, prominent	Medium Thick	solid, heavy
My height is	Above or below average	Average	Average or tall
My muscles are	Wiry, undeveloped	Moderately developed	Solid, stocky, well developed
My weight is	Below average, I lose weight easily	Medium, able to lose or gain weight	Above average, I gain weight easily
Most of my fat is located	Around my waist	Evenly over my body	Around the hips and thighs
My skin is	Dry, flaky, thin, rough, cool to touch	Oily, smooth, with freckles or moles, warm to touch	Oily, thick, smooth, soft to touch
*My complexion is	Dark	Red, ruddy, or yellowish	Pale
*My hair is	Dry, brittle, thin, coarse, brown, black	Fine and straight, blond, red, graying early or balding	Oily, thick, luxuriant, wavy or curly, dark

THE A-Z GUIDE

	VATA	PITTA	KAPHA
My eyebrows are	Thin, dry, and firm	Medium	Thick, large, firm, bushy, oily
My eyes are	Small, nervous, dry, black or brown	Sharp, bright, sensitive to light, gray or green, with a penetrating- gaze	Big, calm, blue, with a loving gaze
My teeth are	Big, crooked or protruding, with thin receding gums	Medium-sized, yellowish and soft, with tender gums	Strong and white with healthy
My nose is	Uneven in shape, small, thin	Long and pointed	Short, round, thick, oily
My lips are	Dry, thin, dark	Soft, pink, red, or yellowish	Oily and smooth, large, thick and firm, pale
My veins are	Prominent	Somewhat visible	Not visible
My shoulders are	Narrow and slope downward	Medium-sized	Broad, firm, developed Wide
My hips are	Narrow	Medium width	Wide

AYURVEDA

	VATA	PITTA	KAPHA
My hands are	Small, dry, cool, with small, long fingers	Medium-sized, moist, warm, pink	Large, oily, cool, firm
My joints are	Thin, small, and make cracking noises	Moderate in size, soft and loose	Large, well lubricated and well knit
My nails are	Dry, rough, brittle, and break easily	Flexible, pink, and lustrous	Thick, smooth, shiny, and hard
My perspiration is	Scanty with no odor	Heavy with strong odor	Moderate or heavy with pleasant odor
My appetite is	Irregular, with skipped meals	Strong, must eat regular meals	Constant, but can skip meals
My sleep pattern is	Irregular, light, interrupted, 5-7 hours a night	Sound and even, 6-8 hours a night	Prolonged and deep, difficult to wake up
My gait is	Quick, short steps	Medium pace, purposeful	Slow and graceful
My energy or endurance is	Low, energy comes in spurts, then need to rest	Well managed	Good, long-lasting

THE A-Z GUIDE

RECORD SHEET

Use this as a permanent record of your test scores to keep track of your doshas.

Baseline VIKRUTI date:	Vata	Pitta	Kapha
Mental-Emotional-Behavioral Symptoms	[ ]	[ ]	[ ]
Physical Symptoms and Illnesses	[ ]	[ ]	[ ]
Total scores	[ ]	[ ]	[ ]

Follow-up VIKRUTI date:	Vata	Pitta	Kapha
Mental-Emotional-Behavioral Symptoms	[ ]	[ ]	[ ]
Physical Symptoms and Illnesses	[ ]	[ ]	[ ]
Total scores	[ ]	[ ]	[ ]

AYURVEDA

Follow-up VIKRUTI date:	Vata	Pitta	Kapha
Mental-Emotional-Behavioral Symptoms	[ ]	[ ]	[ ]
Physical Symptoms and Illnesses	[ ]	[ ]	[ ]
Total scores	[ ]	[ ]	[ ]

PRAKRUTI date: (average scores of three tests)	Vata	Pitta	Kapha
Mental-Emotional-Behavioral Symptoms	[ ]	[ ]	[ ]
Physical Symptoms and Illnesses	[ ]	[ ]	[ ]

THE A-Z GUIDE

Are You Vata, Pitta, or Kapha?

There are ten possible ways to combine the three doshas, known as single-dosha types, two-dosha types, and three dosha types:

Vata
Pitta
Kapha
Vata-Pitta
Pitta-Vata
Vata-Kapha
Kapha-Vata
Pitta-Kapha
Kapha-Pitta
Vata-Pitta-Kapha

The scores from your prakruti test will let you know which combination fits you. If the score for one dosha is much higher than for the second highest—twice as high or higher—you are likely a single-dosha type. Very few people are single-dosha types consisting of pure vata or pitta or kapha. On the other hand if the scores for all the doshas are nearly equal, you are also a rarity—a three dosha type.

More commonly the scores are just about even for two of the doshas. This suggests a two-dosha type, with the person expressing qualities of the two leading doshas nearly equally. However, one dosha still usually predominates, even though it may be slight—thus the fine distinction between pitta-vata and vata-pitta.

If you think of doshas as colors, this principle becomes more understandable. There are three primary colors: blue, red, and yellow. These primary colors combine to form the secondary colors, green (blue-yellow), purple (blue-red), and orange (red-yellow). The primary colors are rarely combined in equal amounts; for example, there are blue-greens (slightly more blue than yellow), reddish purples (with more red than blue), and yellow-orange colors too (containing mostly yellow).

AYURVEDA

In addition the secondary colors usually contain a touch of the third color, allowing for the vast array of colors we see in the world.

Since most people are some combination of all three doshas, at times you will exhibit characteristics of each. Although it's a sign of health to live fully in all three doshas, and to fulfill the most favorable potential that each of them offers, chances are that the strongest part of your nature will bubble up to the surface again and again.

It's important to determine the predominant dosha of your prakruti because that in turn determines the particular Lifestyle Regimen you will be following on a daily basis. However, the doshas shade one another and oftentimes a strong vata imbalance will create confusion. That's because vata leads the other doshas and thus can cause pitta-like or kapha-like symptoms when the underlying cause is really a vata imbalance. Or you may have trouble deciding among the possible answers because aggravated vata brings too much energy into the brain, causing confusion and indecision.

Dr. Vasant Lad, an eminent Ayurvedic clinician and author, offers this prakruti-in-a-nutshell story: Three people walk into an elevator. It gets stuck on the fourth floor. The vata type exclaims, "Oh my God!" and starts trying to force open the door, pressing all the buttons, calling for help. The pitta type yells, "STOP! I've got a plan; you do this, you do that, and I'll try this other thing." Meanwhile the kapha type just sits back and says,

"Let's just wait and see what happens." Which reaction are you most likely to have?

You will also find it helpful to use the following profiles as a supplement to the characteristics provided in the tests to help you pinpoint your dominant dosha. Remember, everyone will exhibit some of the characteristics of each dosha at various times; what's important to focus on is what you are like most of the time.

THE A-Z GUIDE

VATA: Vatas are light, changeable, and unpredictable as the wind. They have a light, thin build; a restless mind and body, and are light sleepers. They move and think quickly, love excitement and change, go to sleep at different times every night, skip meals, and keep irregular habits in general. When in balance, they are cheerful, enthusiastic, resilient, charming, vibrant, vivacious, sensitive, and full of imaginative ideas and creative energy, exhilarated and exhilarating to be around. Imbalanced vata types are worriers, prone to insomnia and constipation. They can be spaced-out, unfocused airheads. They go out of balance most easily and may have started becoming ill in childhood or adolescence.

PITTA: People in whom pitta predominates are intense and fiery, with a strong drive, self-control, and piercing eyes that burn right through you. Of medium build and strength, they exhibit sharp hunger and thirst (pittas get irritable and feel faint if they don't eat on time), and wilt in hot weather. Pitta people communicate through their skin—they blush and flush easily and are radiant when healthy and happy. When in balance, they are joyful, extremely creative, and have an enterprising character that enjoys challenges; they have a sharp intellect and precise, articulate speech. They live by their watches and can't bear waiting or being delayed. Pittas are natural leaders and take command of a situation (or feel that they should). Imbalanced pittas can be annoyingly perfectionist and overly demanding and critical of themselves and others, prone to sarcasm, sharp anger, and irritability under stress. Pittas generally enjoy good health, since their digestion is so strong. However, when out of balance, they are classic type-A personalities, prone to heartburn, ulcers, and heart attacks.

KAPHA: This is the slow, grounded, solid, relaxed dosha. Kapha types are earthy, heavy, with full, gently curving figures or powerful, muscular builds and great endurance; you can find yourself getting lost in their large wide eyes. They act and think methodically—they need a long time to digest information and food and are slow to get out of bed in the morning. When in balance, kaphas are calm, graceful, loving, nurturing, sympathetic, forgiving, and slow to anger. Kaphas, however, seek comfort from eating and tend to obesity and may gain weight just by looking at chocolate cream pie. Their earthiness and steadiness can slide into heaviness of heart and spirit, and a rigid adherence to the status quo. This dosha most strongly feels the need for a strong morning espresso, and may be sluggish in general. Because of its steadiness and inertia, Kapha is least likely to go out of balance and cause ill health.

STEP 3: DETERMINE THE IMBALANCE

Now that you have your two sets of numbers, you are ready to use them to determine where your current imbalance lies, which will guide you in choosing which Ayurvedic practices to follow. This can be confusing for the beginner—and a complex process even for the seasoned Ayurvedic practitioner. However, we have simplified the process so that you really can't go wrong.

The first rule of thumb is: Look at the relationships between the doshas in your vikruti. Is the dosha with the highest score more than 10 points higher than the next highest dosha? If so, this indicates a significant imbalance in the highest dosha, because that is where most of your symptoms are occurring. (Remember, however, we are talking only about your vikruti, not your prakruti. A difference of 10 points in your prakruti is not a sign of imbalance, it is a sign of predominance.) For example let's say your vikruti is vata 45, pitta 30, and kapha 23. Because your vikruti vata is more than 10 points higher than the next highest dosha (pitta), this indicates a vata imbalance.

However, the highest-scoring dosha may not always be the dosha you need to treat directly. This brings us to the next rule: It's highly likely that you will have a vata imbalance, whether or not this is obvious from your scores. That's because vata leads the other doshas. Vata is the energy that directs the nervous system, which is the master switch for all the body systems. That's why so many problems are stress-related, either directly or indirectly. Because of stress your nervous system may be stuck in the "on" position, or be so depleted that it cannot turn on when it is appropriate. When this happens, it can throw the other doshas out of balance too. Depending on the stage of the imbalance, the other doshas

THE A-Z GUIDE

could be either abnormally high or abnormally low. So if either pitta or kapha seems to be out of balance, you can bet the family farm that vata is out of balance too.

The next rule is to consider pitta. Your pitta score is the measure of your digestive fire. Vata leads the doshas, but pitta is responsible for balancing them. Therefore if your fire is too low or too high, it disturbs the levels of vata and kapha.

STEP 4: STABILIZE YOUR DOSHAS

The first thing most people need to do, then, is to stabilize vata and calm down the nervous system to get the neurochemicals to stabilize. Most people will also need to stabilize pitta by rekindling the digestive fire. While this may seem contradictory or confusing, it is not, because calming vata (the leader) helps stabilize pitta; stimulating pitta (the balancer) helps stabilize vata.

To begin, go to Chapter 6 and follow the Daily Lifestyle Regimen that is appropriate for vata. Read through chapters 3, 4, and 5 to understand the Ayurvedic practices that go into the daily regimen, and to learn about the practices that increase the agni (digestive fire), such as the Ten-Day Ginger Treatment. As you'll see, there are a large variety of practices to choose from, and it's not likely you'll adopt all of them for yourself or your family. So after reading through your options, think about the areas that appeal to you most, or that will be- easiest for you to implement.

At first glance changing your diet seems the most logical place to begin to better support your agni. The Ayurvedic diet has gotten a lot of attention, and eating is something that everyone does anyway. So some people find this is the aspect that they can relate to and plug into most easily. However, diet isn't the only thing that affects the doshas—and it may not even be the most important thing. That's why although you need to pay attention to what you eat, we feel it's a shame that people put so much emphasis on diet as a cure-all. In the process they forget there are other senses besides taste, and they bypass other practices, especially

AYURVEDA

those involving their emotional lives. They think that if they eat right and get enough exercise, they'll be fine. But we find in our practice that some of the best-fed, well-exercised people have the worst emotional lives and mental states. Remember there's much more to life and to Ayurveda than diet, so avoid becoming obsessive about food or addicted to a particular diet.

Instead of changing your diet right away, you might want to do what we often recommend for our patients: Save your dietary changes for later and start your vata-stabilizing program with the general Lifestyle Recommendations—the oil massage, vata tea, yoga, and meditation—all of which are included in Chapter 3. That way you're not dealing with such a loaded subject as food, and instead of taking something away, you're adding some things that are pleasurable.

Once you have established a basic lifestyle routine of things you will do every day, you're ready to fine-tune your program. Turn to the A–Z section and pick one or two symptoms that trouble you the most— usually those that are severe, frequent, and consistent. Zero in on them by adding the more specific remedies from chapters 4 and 5 recommended for those conditions. For example you may also add one of the churnas (special combinations of herbs and spices) and an aromatherapy from Chapter 5.

STEP 5: MONITOR YOUR PROGRESS

Follow the general balancing practices and symptom-specific remedies until the symptoms subside. Depending on the condition and how deep-seated it is, this may take a year or more. Be sure to monitor your progress by repeating the vikruti test every three months. The goal is to have the ratios among the vikruti doshas come close to those in your prakruti.

THE A-Z GUIDE

STEP 6: MAINTAIN BALANCE

When the test shows that the ratios of the doshas in your vikruti have come close to those in your prakruti, cut back to just the general practices in your Lifestyle Regimen tailored for the dosha that predominates in your prakruti. If old symptoms should return or new ones appear, add to your daily regimen the specific remedies recommended for those conditions in the A—Z section.

EXAMPLES

Paulina: Paulina is a copy editor who often works under pressure of a deadline. Adding to her stress level, she recently separated from her husband of fifteen years. Paulina's initial vikruti scores were:

Vata: 22 (mental) + 15 (physical) = 37 total

Pitta: 14 (mental) + 19 (physical) = 33 total

Kapha: 11 (mental) + 7 (physical) = 18 total

Her prakruti scores were:

Vata: 29 (mental) + 15 (physical) — 44 total

Pitta: 36 (mental) + 51 (physical) = 87 total

Kapha: 7 (mental) + 10 (physical) = 17 total

Paulina's pitti in her prakruti is nearly twice as high as her vata, making her a pitta type. But these two doshas are nearly even in her vikruti, indicating an aggravated vata.

An Ayurvedic practitioner would say that Paulina's vata is pushing her pitta, or that the vata wind is blowing out the pitta fire. Her nervous system, ruled by vata, is hyperactive and sending messages all over her body, suppressing the pitta and her transformative energy. As a result her

AYURVEDA

agni or digestive fires are low and not digesting food, thoughts, emotions; and ama (toxins) is starting to develop in the system.

Since vata leads the other doshas and the nervous system runs all the other systems, Paulina needs to calm and restore her nervous system. The ideal is to bring her current vata down to about half of her pitta so that the ratio is closer to that in her prakruti. To restore the balance, she should follow a vata-stabilizing daily regimen, which includes meditation, oil massage, vata tea, and yoga.

She also needs to increase her digestive fires, which she does by doing the Ten-Day Ginger Treatment at the beginning of every month, and by adding summer churna to her food at least once a day. She then looks at the A–Z section to find a couple of symptoms that bother her most— insomnia, fatigue syndrome, and indigestion—and adds specific remedies to take care of those.

Rosemary: Next, we look at Rosemary, a woman in her mid-thirties who works for a nonprofit organization. Her vikruti scores were:

Vata: 33 (mental) + 23 (physical) = 56 total
Pitta: 18 (mental) + 17 (physical) = 35 total
Kapha: 13 (mental) + 21 (physical) = 34 total

Her prakruti scores were:

Vata: 25 (mental) + 25 (physical) = 50 total
Pitta: 23 (mental) + 31 (physical) = 54 total
Kapha: 12 (mental) + 9 (physical) = 21 total

In assessing the prakruti scores, Rosemary's pitta is slightly higher than her vata, making her a pitta-vata. But in the vikruti, her vata is much higher than her pitta in her vikruti, indicating an aggravated vata. In applying the first rule of thumb, we see that her pitta and kapha are much too low. Rosemary's vata imbalance is accompanied by a low digestive fire; she also has a lubrication problem because kapha is also too low. She is bothered by anxiety and fear and recurrent vaginitis, which are vata-related. She also complains of procrastination (it took her several weeks to get around to completing this self-assessment). This is a classic kapha imbalance, but an Ayurvedic practitioner would say that in her case it is being driven by the vata aggravation, which dries out the oils, getting her stuck. Her tissues are getting malnourished and dried out; this would indicate osteoporosis in an older woman, and a high risk of osteoporosis in later life for this thirty-three-year-old. Rosemary needs to follow an Ayurvedic program for two to three years to slow and prevent the progression of this serious condition.

Simply stated, she needs to calm down her vata, get her fire going and lubricate her mind and tissues. In addition to following the vata-balancing Daily Lifestyle Regimen, she adds vata aromatherapy, which is especially good because aromas don't need to pass through the digestive system—they go directly to her mind to provide the lubrication it needs. She drinks vata tea and uses winter churna every day for three to six months. She adds the Ten-Day Ginger Treatment once a month to get her fire up. She also drinks one cup of kapha tea every other day to get her kapha going again and stop it from weighing down her pitta; to the tea she adds 1/4 teaspoon trikatu, a concentrated combination herbal remedy that further increases her digestive fire.

Allen: Finally, let's look at Allen, a graphic designer in his late forties: His vikruti scores were:

Vata: 18 (mental) + 9 (physical) = 27 total
Pitta: 17 (mental) + 9 (physical) = 26 total
Kapha: 13 (mental) + 18 (physical) = 31 total

His prakruti scores were:

Vata: 35 (mental) + 24 (physical) = 59 total
Pitta: 30 (mental) + 38 (physical) = 68 total
Kapha: 25 (mental) + 30 (physical) = 55 total

The vikruti scores show that this man does not have an overwhelming imbalance, since there is less than a 10-point difference among the doshas. However, his prakruti shows that his pitta is high, indicating that it's his nature to have a lot of pitta energy—an energy that is not reflected in his vikruti. This indicates that his pitta is being suppressed. We also notice that his vata is somewhat low in his vikruti and his kapha is elevated, compared with his prakruti. His most bothersome and consistent symptoms are allergies (a pitta imbalance), confusion (vata), and a struggle with overweight (usually a kapha problem, but in Allen's case, the other two doshas are also involved). An Ayurvedic practitionerwould tell him that in spite of his weight problems and lethargy, he's not as "kaphic" as he thinks he is—he has more energy and is more dynamic than he seems. Somewhere in his childhood his ama got clogged and his ambition got clogged along with it. His mind-body has learned to hold back his passion, but if he got his fire up, he could express this creative energy more freely.

Once again, since vata leads the doshas, Allen needs to stabilize his vata by following the vata daily regimen and drinking vata tea first thing in the morning. However, to deal with his weight problem, he should eat kapha rather than vata foods—he needs to avoid pasta, rice, and pastries and emphasize high-enzyme foods such as mango, papaya, and pineapple. To stimulate his pitta, he should eat fresh grated ginger every day, and once a month he needs to really pump up the volume by doing the Ten-Day Ginger Treatment.

THE A-Z GUIDE

AYURVEDA AND YOUR CHILD

What makes your baby tick? Does she sleep a lot, is she always on the go, or is she happier staying home and calmly watching her mobile? Does she get gas easily, does she have a tantrum if her diaper isn't changed right away, or do you constantly have to check on her because she is content and quiet? Is she roly-poly or does she have a slight build? Is she easygoing or aggressive, does she tend to be fearful or aggravated? Does she avidly follow everything with her eyes; or does she just smile sweetly and go back to thinking her cosmic baby thoughts?

Observing your baby and understanding his or her doshas gives you a more effective way of responding to his or her unique individual way of being and a new tolerance for the things you don't understand. By determining whether your baby is predominantly vata, pitta, or kapha, you acquire new tools and technology to help you guide your baby to balance before any deep imbalances set in and frustrate your baby as well as you the parent.

The first thing to understand is that infancy and childhood are considered to be the kapha time of life for physical and emotional development. The emotional characteristics of this dosha include being easygoing and contented; if it loses its balance, kapha becomes possessive, depressed, and stubborn. Next look at the chart below and determine the prakruti of your baby. Every two months or so review the chart and see how the emotional, behavioral, and physical patterns develop.

Vata Babies . . .
> take short sleeps
> may tend toward constipation
> appear very alert
> move their eyes a lot
> have delicate nerves and jump at loud noises
> like lively, soft music

AYURVEDA

Pitta Babies . . .

    have a reddish complexion

    have penetrating eyes

    get fussy when hungry

    are impatient when their needs aren't met quickly

    are interested in everything

    don't want to leave when people are around

Kapha Babies . . .

    sleep easily

    smile a lot

    are content

    have long, slow eye movements

    do not move around much

Vata Toddlers . . .

    are busy, busy, busy

    have active imaginations

    are happy to be alone and be in a fantasy world

    do not like loud, fast noises

    do not like naps

    fidget and move a lot

    eat lots of small meals

    like to participate, but feel intimidated by lead roles

Pitta Toddlers . . .

    are creative

    like to play in groups and lead the games

    eat good meals, get cranky if eating is delayed

    get rashes easily

    may have food allergies and sensitivities

    get frustrated easily, but forget about it fast and move on to the next enterprise

    play intensely, then crash for a nap, which reenergizes them

    like to do important jobs and will do them expertly

Kapha Toddlers . . .

    participate joyously

    are observers, not leaders

THE A-Z GUIDE

remember every fact and will repeat them to you if asked
can play for a long time without a nap
are basically very contented
if out of balance, are possessive with toys and with Mom and Dad

The most important gift you can give your baby each day is the gift of sesame oil massage (this is called abhyanga and is more fully described in Chapter 3). This massage is the foundation of good health for the rest of your baby's life. It not only increases circulation and strengthens immune function, but it encourages a close, endearing relationship between mother, father, and baby, and as a result your baby will become more relaxed and emotionally satisfied. Start this simple, beautiful practice after the umbilical cord falls off. Do the massage at the same time every day, and exercise your baby afterward. You may feed your baby a half hour afterward.

CHAPTER THREE
THE FUNDAMENTAL PRACTICES OF AYURVEDA

In this chapter we provide you with a basic guide to the daily general Ayurvedic practices that form the foundation for maintaining, creating, or restoring good health. They are based on the observation that everything you eat, do, or come into contact with influences the doshas. Once you understand your unique doshic mind-body balance, you can tailor your daily lifestyle so that it includes the powerful disease-preventive practices, described in this chapter, that celebrate your strengths, strengthen your weaknesses, and support agni, the digestive fire on which health is based. The practices are part of the daily routines recommended in Chapter 6; you can use them either individually or along with some of the other practices and specific therapies described in chapters 4 and 5.

THE A-Z GUIDE

VITALITY, LONGEVITY, AND SPIRITUAL AND MENTAL HEALTH

Ayurveda recognizes that your unique genetic code includes both strengths and weaknesses, and that your ability to resist disease and the rate at which we age may be in part genetic. But much of disease and aging depends on lifestyle, attitude, and environmental factors. Ayurveda teaches that the mind-body is self-regulating and self-healing and that certain practices clear away obstacles that get in the way of health and healing. Every day you can choose habits that are harmful and wearing on the system—and thus increase the risk of physical and mental disease, premature and decrepit aging, and untimely death. Or you can choose ways that are protective and rejuvenating—and thus help prevent disease, slow aging, and increase longevity. The Ayurvedic lifestyle is a way to choose the second path, a life full of vitality and spiritual and mental health until the very end.

Although conventional medicine is paying increasing attention to disease prevention, rejuvenation is often overlooked. Ayurveda recognizes the importance of rejuvenating your mind-body and advocates certain practices that take your well-fed, rested body to the next level, wherein your physiology is producing physiological bliss and its by-product, ojas. In this chapter we not only recommend general lifestyle practices and eating patterns but we also teach you how to do oiling and cleansing practices called pancha karma. These are rejuvenation practices that may be done every day. Pancha karma techniques help you rid your body of toxic chemicals in the air, water, and food, and of toxic emotional stresses that debilitate the nervous system; they keep your body clean so that it can absorb nutrients and deeply relax and strengthen the whole system. In these various ways they thus revitalize the tissues to help delay aging and promote longevity.

Ayurveda recognizes the interdependence of body, mind, and spirit. Meditation and yoga are the two closely related practices that work on the spiritual and mental planes (yoga also works on the physical plane). They are particularly useful for people who want to delve more deeply

AYURVEDA

into Ayurveda and themselves. Spiritual and mental practices are the heart and soul of Ayurveda, and although teaching them in depth is beyond the scope of this book, in this chapter we provide you with a simple meditation technique and discuss the benefits and roles meditation and yoga play in disease prevention, mental and spiritual vitality, and longevity.

GENERAL LIFESTYLE RECOMMENDATIONS

1. Get the right amount of sleep. In Ayurveda proper sleep is paramount because it promotes mental digestion of everything you took in that day. Both the amount and the timing matter. In general you should be up before the sun rises and asleep by ten P.M. in order to take advantage of your body's natural rhythms and functions. (Please turn to Chapter 6 for a discussion of how our body rhythms change with the hours of the day and the seasons of the year.)

2. Pay attention to elimination. In Ayurveda it is important to have at least one bowel movement every day, in the morning. Don't ignore the urge when you have to go, because elimination of waste products reduces the accumulation of ama. One of the wonderful things about Ayurveda is that its practices bring about regularity, without the need for the strong laxative jolt of coffee in the morning.

3. Avoid suppressing any natural urges, including sneezes, thirst, hunger, coughs, yawns, tears, laughter, runny nose, flatus, feces, and urine. Ayurveda believes suppression can lead to diseases later on.

4. Love, happiness, and clarity in our relationships and everyday life are important to good health and long life.

5. Get out in the fresh air and sunlight every day for at least twenty minutes. Take a walk, sit outdoors when you eat lunch. Being

around nature is a traditional Ayurvedic prescription, and recent studies support the observation that nature is good for your health.

6.   Sip water throughout the day. Most beneficial is to drink pure spring water or filtered water that has been boiled for ten minutes. Let the water cool to room temperature and sip one or two ounces every half hour to restore balance to your bioenergetic body. This practice of drinking bioenergetically treated water is inexpensive, easy, and very powerful for balancing all three doshas. The boiling is not for the purpose of purifying the water but rather because it is an energetic treatment. Boiling creates movement, which stimulates vata; it creates heat, which stimulates pitta; and it creates steam, which stimulates kapha.

7.   Clean your tongue, not just your teeth. After you have cleaned your teeth in the morning, scrape the ama from your tongue every day. It is preferable that vatas use a gold tongue-scraper, pittas use silver, and kaphas use copper (for suppliers, see the "Resources" section of this book). A stainless steel scraper is acceptable for everyone. There are also plastic tongue scrapers available at pharmacies, or you can simply use your toothbrush to use forward-moving strokes beginning at the back of the tongue to remove the morning residue coating your tongue. Be careful not to scrape too far back on your tongue, or you will trigger the gag reflex. Scraping is said to stimulate the digestive fire and also remove bacteria from your tongue.

8.   Use television prudently, if at all. Television can have a negative or a positive effect, depending how you use it. For example there are many healing and educational videotapes available. You can learn yoga from a videotape, or you can heal an illness, as chronicled by Norman Cousins in his classic book, *Anatomy of an Illness*. But watching too much increases vata because it stimulates your sight and hearing, and increases kapha because of its passive nature. Watching shows that are violent or frightening and full of negative

emotions may make a subtle impression on the dosha associated with those emotions.

9. Sex: Ayurveda believes that sex is a wonderful part of life and can enhance spirituality. Generally it is thought that having sexual relations twice a week is healthy, but everyone should obey his or her natural urges while in a balanced state.

DIET AND EATING HABITS

Eating Ayurvedically is healthful because it provides a diet of balanced amounts of carbohydrate, protein, and fat and is rich in nutrient-dense fresh fruits and vegetables and whole grains. But in Ayurveda food is more than fuel to keep you going, more than a bunch of chemicals that supply essential vitamins and minerals. Wholesome food is a total experience that can nourish you emotionally as well as physically.

The following Ayurvedic recommendations are designed to help make food nourishing in every way. They are based on ancient observations and insights. Perhaps most profound is the concept that all foods and beverages are imprinted with a vital memory. It remembers its whole life and, through its DNA, it also harbors remembrances of its ancestors' lives. Food passes this rich store of knowledge to you when you eat it, providing a form of energy that connects it and you to other people and to the earth. Food that is organically grown, raised on small local farms, and lovingly prepared carries more positive, nourishing energy (prana) than food that is degraded and adulterated, raised with artificial chemicals, and impersonally grown on factory farms. If your natural urge to have such positive emotional connections remains unfulfilled, you may try to get satisfaction by overeating or acquiring an excess of material things.

A related concept is the idea that specific doshas have an affinity for certain tastes (more about the role of the six tastes—sweet, salty, sour,

THE A-Z GUIDE

bitter, pungent, and astringent— in Chapter 5). Certain tastes aggravate doshas, and other tastes stabilize them. Food has other qualities as well— heavy or light, hot or cool, dry or moist—that affect the doshas. We need the proper combinations of all these qualities in our food to remain in balance. The timing of meals is also believed to affect digestion, since your body goes through natural cycles of digestion and assimilation of food and elimination of waste. Keep these ideas about food in mind as you follow the following basic principles:

1. Eat pure, fresh, local, unprocessed foods during their natural season of growth. Depending on the dosha you are aiming to stabilize, emphasize or reduce the quantity of certain foods you eat, as recommended in the food charts. Since you will be eating locally grown food, you need to make adjustments in some categories. No food, however, is completely off-limits; if you are a vata type, it doesn't mean you never eat an apple, or that pittas can never have corn again, or that double-fudge brownies will never touch a kapha's lips. You can eat anything occasionally.

2. Shop at health food stores and farmers' markets—or grow some of your own food. Avoid food that has been adulterated with pesticides, synthetic preservatives, and hormones. (Especially avoid commercial cow's milk, meat, and poultry, which are produced under stressful conditions for the animals and thus contain many negative memories, which are passed on to you when you eat them.)

3. Minimize or avoid foods in the nightshade family. These include tomatoes, eggplant, peppers, and white potatoes. They contain chemicals called solanines, which cause nervous system disorders; they also dehydrate the joints and thus worsen arthritis. If you do eat these foods, use turmeric to lessen the detrimental effects.

4. Sip warm or hot water before or during meals to aid digestion, but avoid icy or cold drinks before or with meals because they cool the digestive fire.

AYURVEDA

5. Following a vegetarian diet as closely as possible is not only spiritually healthier, it's physiologically healthier. The Ayurvedic tradition recommends eating light foods; now modern scientific studies are supporting this age-old way of eating to prevent many diseases including cancer and heart disease. Heavy foods such as meat stress the system, and you can get all the protein you need from vegetables, grains, and beans.

6. Milk is considered to be one of the most important foods in Ayurveda. But if you drink it, it must be organic and come from cows raised under gentle conditions. Milk is only to be taken cooked and along with specific spices good for your dosha—not cold and straight out of the refrigerator. If you are allergic to cow's milk, you may substitute soy, rice, or nut milks.

7. Although some people require sweet foods, this means naturally sweet (fruits, grains, some vegetables such as carrots and sweet potatoes), which should still be eaten in moderation. Avoid refined sugar of all kinds; and use natural sweeteners in moderation, as appropriate to your dosha, such as honey, molasses, or Sucanat (a new product that is made of dehydrated juice of organic sugar cane).

8. Oils are an important source of internal lubrication in Ayurveda. Vata, the driest dosha, has the least amount of lubrication and requires the most oil from food. Pittas have intense, hot body oils and need less oil from food. Kaphas also have plenty of oils and need the least amount of outside oils. In most cases use non hydrogenated, unrefined, cold-pressed oils sold at health food stores and Indian and Oriental food stores. Ghee, or clarified butter, is also recommended in cooking and for flavoring. In experiments conducted at Ohio State University, the small amounts traditionally used (about 1 teaspoon per day) did not raise cholesterol.

9. Avoid alcohol and coffee in general and especially with meals.

THE A-Z GUIDE

10. Eat foods that work together in combination. Avoid the following combinations because when eaten together these foods create poor digestion, malabsorption, and clogging of the channels:

   - Melons . . . . .with any other food
   - Sour fruits . . . . . .with milk or yogurt
   - Bananas . . . . with milk, corn, starches, or radishes
   - Fish . . . . .with milk or yogurt
   - Meat . . . . .with milk, yogurt, or eggs
   - Cheese . . . . .with yogurt, eggs, or mango
   - Bread . . . . .with milk
   - Eggs . . . . .with milk, yogurt, starches
   - Starches . . . . .with yogurt, dates, persimmons, or milk
   - Raisins . . . . .with radishes or corn
   - Cucumbers . . . . . .with mango, lemon, potato, eggplant, or tomatoes
   - Tomatoes . . . . .with lemon, milk or yogurt
   - Potatoes . . . . .with milk or yogurt
   - Eggplant . . . . .with milk or yogurt

11. Most people are in the habit of eating much more food than they really need. Each meal should consist of about two and a half handfuls of food so that after a meal your stomach contains one-third solid food, one-third liquid, and one-third remains empty to allow space and energy for digestion.

12. To facilitate complete digestion, eat your main meal at lunchtime; eat a light supper several hours before you plan to go to sleep.

13. Eat meals at about the same time every day if possible. This is especially important for calming excess vata. However, it is best to eat food on an empty stomach; wait until your last meal has been digested, no matter what the clock says.

AYURVEDA

14. Don't rush, read, stand up, and watch TV, drive, or have excited conversation while eating. Focus on the food, chew food well, and take time to enjoy every mouthful so that you consciously and unconsciously take in the memory that food imparts and so that your mind-body can assimilate the nutrients. But don't make the meal a drawn-out affair.

15. Don't eat while you are upset; wait until you have calmed down.

16. Prepare food so that it is tasty, pleasant to look at, and eaten in pleasant surroundings. Refer to Appendix D for Ayurvedic cookbooks.

17. According to Ayurveda, the thoughts and emotions you have while handling food become part of your food. If you're angry or tense while preparing food, that's the energy you are taking in and feeding to other people. So cook with positive emotions, such as love and kindness toward the food you are about to eat or share with others. In addition when possible, use simple, nonmotorized hand tools to prepare food: The more your own hands come into contact with food, the more opportunity for the food's energy to mix with yours, and the closer you feel to food and the earth from which it comes.

18. Don't eat microwaved foods, because according to Ayurveda they have had their life force destroyed.

19. Most food should be warm or hot—or at least room temperature— and usually cooked. Never sleep right after eating—make sure you leave a few hours in between. Rest after lunch by lying down on your left side for a few minutes, and take a short walk in the evening after dinner.

THE A-Z GUIDE

EXERCISE

In spite of the so-called fitness boom, we are a sedentary nation. According to a 1996 Surgeon General's Report, only 29 percent of adult Americans get regular vigorous or sustained exercise. Many adults—and children—have become couch potatoes (and the increasing use of computers may make us even more physically inactive). Exercise has been shown to improve lung function; burn fat; increase stamina; reduce risk of coronary heart disease, stroke, osteoporosis, diabetes, and possibly many types of cancer; lower blood pressure; help reduce stress and anxiety; work better than psychotherapy for depression; and improve resistance to disease. In Ayurveda, exercise is recognized as good preventive medicine because it also enables more prana (life energy) to reach the tissues by cleaning and clearing all channels, promoting circulation and excretion of wastes. Recent studies suggest that exercise doesn't have to be torture, or take up all our free time, in order to do us good. Instead of prescribing intense workouts done for at least thirty minutes three to five times a week, the newest recommendations are that moderate exercise can be beneficial. And that short periods of everyday activities and chores such as raking leaves, walking, dancing, gardening, and playing with the kids can accumulate and be as beneficial as an equivalent amount of time spent working out.

Ayurveda has long advocated a moderate approach to exercise. It warns you not to overdo it, because this could shorten life span and lower resistance to disease. In Ayurveda the rule of thumb is to avoid spending more than half your energy on exercise; so if an hour of running exhausts you, don't run for more than half an hour at a time. The exertion level should be just enough to cause you to sweat on your forehead, under your arms, and along your spinal column—this is the level at which activity stimulates agni, relaxes you, and helps you sleep, and at which sweating reduces toxins, burns fat, and elevates mood by producing endorphins. But beware of becoming addicted to endorphins (your body's natural morphine), a habit that is especially common in vata types.

AYURVEDA

It's also wise to tailor your exercise program to your prakruti. For example, vata types tend to prefer the most vigorous workouts, but they get exhausted if they exercise too strenuously for too long. They do well with slow, low-intensity exercises such as medium-paced walking, yoga, dancing, and tai chi. People who are predominantly pitta, the fiery dosha, do well with competitive sports and steady, medium-intensity exercises such as hiking, particularly in natural settings containing the colors green and blue, as well as cooling activities such as swimming. Kapha, the lethargic dosha, needs vigorous, stimulating workouts such as aerobic dance, jogging and running, and weight training five or six times a week. Everyone should walk and do yoga. And if possible, everyone should exercise early in the morning to balance the -morning's predominantly kapha-esque, slow-moving characteristics.

OIL MASSAGE (ABHYANGA)

Oil massage is one of the several purification techniques collectively known as pancha karma. In India massage is a natural part of daily life. Infants are massaged every day from the day they are born to age three, and weekly after that. By age six, children are massaging their elders. It's common for entire families to massage one another once a week. Pregnant women are massaged daily during pregnancy and for more than a month after giving birth. Sensual massage with aphrodisiac oils is advised in treatises on sexology.

In Ayurveda, bathing is a ritual designed to clean you inside and out, and begins with the application of oil. Applying oil to your skin lubricates, protects, detoxifies, and rejuvenates your skin and nervous system, while soothing your endocrine system. The oil helps loosen and liquify ama so that the toxins can drain into the body's gastrointestinal tract for elimination. It is an excellent antidote for modern stresses and is said to help you achieve the balance that is the foundation of spiritual development. As the body's largest and most sensitive organ, your skin deserves abhyanga every day. In Ayurveda getting a massage or giving one to yourself is one of the most effective and pleasant ways you can balance vata and is a wonderful way to start the day. With regular

THE A-Z GUIDE

practice you'll see why abhyanga is considered to be the crown jewel of rejuvenation, prevention, and longevity.

Sesame oil is recommended for vata, pitta, and kapha types, and for healthy people as well as those suffering from an illness. The only exception is when your kapha is aggravated—in this case you should use a dry massage, described below. Be sure to get cold-pressed organic oil from a health food store. Olive oil is also acceptable, and coconut oil works well for pitta types. Never use mineral oil or any other oil that is not digestible (the skin is a digestive organ). It's traditional to cook the oil one time, heating it until it forms tiny bubbles. This is said to cure the oil and prevent it from turning rancid. Certain conditions respond best to medicated oils—oils to which special herbs and fragrant spices have been added, as specified in the A–Z section. Once you've been treating yourself to abhyanga regularly, it's hard to stop, and even busy people manage to make time.

"If I get lazy or pressed for time and skip my daily abhyanga, I really start to miss it. I feel scattered, less grounded, and less able to cope. I love the little pool of serenity it creates in the morning . . . a quiet, sensual time just for myself before I get swept up in the madness of the day. I think what a different world it would be if everyone had a sesame oil massage in the morning."

How to Do Self-Massage

We have found that while patients used to balk at doing self-massage, this is no longer the case. Today my frazzled patients welcome setting aside this special time in the morning just for themselves. And it's even nicer if you can exchange massages with someone. Abhyanga can take as few as ten minutes, or up to twenty minutes if you work slowly and take your time. If you are pressed for time, you can do a mini-massage instead of the full-body massage; this involves just the ears, feet, and forehead. If you perform abhyanga regularly, you'll never have to spend time and money applying "moisturizing" skin creams.

AYURVEDA

To begin, warm the oil (slightly less than 1/4 cup is enough for the whole body) to skin temperature or slightly warmer to make the massage more pleasant. Ne way is to use a small ceramic cup placed on an electric coffee warmer; you may also put the oil in a small dish or container and set that in a bowl of hot water until it reaches skin temperature. Be careful not to make the oil too hot, to avoid burning and scalding. Begin at the top of your body and work your way down, and do about twenty strokes on each part of your body, as described below.

First apply a thin coat all over your body to maximize the amount of time the oil comes into contact with your skin. Then massage your face, ears, and back of the ears, using short, vigorous strokes. It is traditional to apply oil to your scalp as well, but I personally have found this strips my hair of body. If you have little or no hair or wash your hair every day, this may not be a problem; alternatively you can give your scalp an invigorating oil-free massage instead. Proceed to your neck and shoulders, using your fingers and the flat of your hand. Then massage your upper arms and lower arms, using long back and-forth strokes. Use a circular motion for the joints, including your shoulders. Massage your chest and abdomen using a clockwise motion. Next massage your hip joints, buttocks, legs, and then the soles of your feet.

The oil is usually left on while you do some light exercise, such as yoga, and then washed off in bath or shower with warm water; use mild soap, but only on the body parts that really need it. In India people chant mantras or sing devotional songs while bathing, which, according to Ayurvedic scholar Robert Svoboda, "makes the bath or shower water into a vehicle for those vibrations and transports their purifying power into the deepest levels of being." Whether you chant or sing or not, be careful to avoid slipping on the oil. Leaving a thin film of the oil on the body is said to be beneficial.

THE A-Z GUIDE

DRY MASSAGE (GARSHANA)

If you are a kapha type or your kapha is aggravated, give yourself an invigorating thy massage every day instead of an oil massage. Follow the directions for abhyanga, above, using silk gloves designed for dry body rubs and sold at bath shops. You can easily make a simple mitt from a piece of silk that you have folded over and sewn to form a pocket. You may also use chickpea flour, available at health food stores; rub this on your skin with the silk gloves or your bare hands. This may also be done two or three times a week by everyone, and followed with the oil massage.

NASAL-PASSAGE LUBRICATION (NASAYA)

Modern allergists tell us we inhale two and a half tablespoons of solid particles every day! Car exhaust, smog, formaldehyde fumes, pollens, and more effortlessly enter your nose and irritate the delicate nerve endings of your nasal passages and eventually end up in your lungs. Nasaya is a very simple technique that will clean your sinuses, lubricate and protect the tender tissues responsible for your sense of smell, and improve your voice. Once or twice a day insert one or two drops of sesame oil into your nose, using either an eyedropper or the tip of your little finger; inhale strongly so that the oil is carried into your nasal passages. Plain sesame oil used alone works wonders as a general protectant; there are also specific herbal oils and medicated ghees used to correct imbalances of the eyes, ears, nose, and throat that we recommend for specific conditions in the A—Z section of this book.

BREATHING PRACTICES (PRANAYAMA)

Breathing exercises are a part of the discipline of yoga and are said to help balance consciousness, improve creativity, and allow us to feel joy, bliss, peace, and love. Ayurveda recommends that special attention be paid to breathing because prana, the vital life force, enters the body with each

AYURVEDA

breath. Traditionally these exercises are done while sitting comfortably cross-legged on the floor; if you want to use this position, you should elevate your sitting bones with a large folded towel or two or a meditation cushion. Loose-fitting, comfortable clothes and dark, quiet surroundings also help, but are not required. You can do these breathing practices anywhere, anytime you need to "take five," during a yoga practice, or as a prelude to meditation.

Abdominal Breathing

Most people take only shallow breaths and fill only the top part of the lungs. But the nerves in this part of the lung are there to deal with a stress response and they trigger the body to produce stress hormones, which are harmful when prolonged. By way of contrast the lower lobes of the lungs contain nerves that calm and regenerate the body. This simple technique teaches you to fill the whole lung with air, massaging the internal organs and reducing anxiety, depression, nervousness, muscle tension, and fatigue. It may also pave the way for your entering the "alpha state," in which the mind is exceptionally calm and clear.

1. To begin, sit or lie down in a comfortable position. Rest one hand over your abdomen and one on your upper chest. Take a few slow breaths and notice where your breath goes—does your chest rise and fall but not your abdomen? Or does your abdomen move alone? Which rises or falls first?

2. Next breathe in slowly through your nose, attempting to fill your abdomen first, by lowering your diaphragm. This may take several tries for some people. Imagine your abdomen is a balloon.

3. Once your abdomen is filled, keep inhaling and fill your chest, allowing it to rise.

4. Exhale slowly through your mouth, first emptying your chest and then your abdomen.

THE A-Z GUIDE

5. Repeat the inhalation and exhalation, trying to slow the breath even more. This should feel like a wave of air, rhythmically entering and leaving your body.

Only inhaling should require any effort. Allow the air to flow out on its own as you let the weight of your chest and abdomen relax down. Try to remember to breathe this way as you go about your everyday activities, as you do yoga, and as you do any type of physical activity. You'll find you'll have more energy and endurance and greater mental clarity.

Alternate-Nostril Breathing

Your nostrils alternate periods of activity during the day. During certain times the left nostril is more active; prana entering the body through this nostril cools and calms you down; during other times the right nostril predominates, and prana entering during this time heats you up. The purpose of alternating nostrils, as instructed below, is to stabilize vata. To cool and balance pitta, breathe in only through the left nostril and breathe out through the right; to heat and stimulate kapha, inhale through the right nostril only and exhale through the left. For best results use abdominal breathing, for the inhalations and exhalations.

1. Using your right hand, place your thumb next to your right nostril and your middle finger next to your left nostril. Gently but firmly close off your right nostril with your thumb. Inhale through your left nostril, bringing your awareness to your heart.

2. Release your right nostril and close off your left nostril with your middle finger, exhaling through your right nostril.

3. Keeping your left nostril closed, inhale through your right nostril.

4. Close off your right nostril and inhale through your left nostril.

5. Repeat this breathing pattern twelve times.

AYURVEDA

MEDITATION

Meditation has traditionally been integral to many cultures and religions around the world, from Roman Catholicism to Jewish mysticism to Tibetan Buddhism. It is as varied as these religions and cultures are themselves, and has many goals, techniques, and effects. Meditation allows mental chatter to quiet and eventually cease, at first for moments and then, with practice, for minutes at a time. During those moments the consciousness and the body are cleansed and you experience the state of pure being, of oneness with the universe—transcendence. Many people find that with regular meditation they experience a profound shift in their inner lives. This in turn can also affect physical health.

In fact hundreds of meditators have been studied and their physiological processes have been measured. Researchers found that meditation.. .

- Reduces blood levels of stress hormones, which are associated with poor health and aging
- Reduces levels of lactate, a substance related to high levels of anxiety
- Lowers or normalizes blood pressure and pulse rate
- Lowers respiration, oxygen consumption, and metabolic rate
- Lowers abnormally high cholesterol levels
- Enhances immune system response
- Increases alpha brain-wave activity, which is present during times of creativity and relaxation
- May increase concentration, memory, and creativity
- Is deeply relaxing and rejuvenating

Some long-term meditators have been found to be five to twelve years younger biologically than they are chronologically, as indicated by their blood pressure, visual acuity, and hearing. New research shows that meditators have up to nearly 50 percent higher levels of a hormone called DHEA. Low levels of DHEA are considered to be a marker for exposure to chronic stress and for aging. High levels of DHEA are

THE A-Z GUIDE

associated with reduced incidence of disorders such as heart disease, breast cancer, and osteoporosis, to name a few.

There are many schools of meditation, but what they all have in common is that they bring your attention to rhythmic breathing, to an object, or to a word or thought or mantra such as the word om. Or you focus outward on something, such as a candle, a picture, God, or a space four feet in front of your nose. The process gently draws you inward until you reach your mind's own deepest nature. Meditation is a different experience for each person, and each session is different as well. The following exercise will help you get a glimpse of what meditation feels like.

If you want to know more or explore this practice more deeply, there are many books and tapes devoted to all kinds of relaxation and meditation techniques (see Appendix B), and excellent teachers in nonsectarian disciplines such as mindfulness and Transcendental Meditation. We encourage you to experiment. Although the study of a meditation system does not necessarily involve adaptation of a religion, there is quite a bit of ritual, faith, and aesthetic variation among the forms. You can get a good feel for whether a particular form is good for you by glancing at the literature, talking to the people involved, or visiting a meeting or ceremony.

How to Meditate

Before beginning choose a word or phrase to bring your attention to, such as the ancient Sanskrit mantra Ham Sah, which means "I am that"; or repeat "five-four-three-two-one" to yourself, or "I am love, I am joy, I am one." If you learn from a teacher you may ask for a mantra known to resonate specifically with your dominant dosha, which enhances meditation's ability to purify the mind and balance the body. Traditionally these mantras are repeated 108 times, using prayer beads to keep track of the repetitions; this is the equivalent of about four or five minutes. Most people start out meditating for twenty minutes—and even that short amount of time can be a challenge. As you go deeper into

AYURVEDA

this practice, you will find the time just flies by and you will want to meditate for thirty or forty-five minutes.

1. Sit in a comfortable position that you can hold for at least twenty minutes, in a quiet place where you won't be disturbed by the phone or other people. A traditional posture is to sit cross-legged on the floor, sitting bones elevated by a meditation cushion (one or more folded-over towels can substitute).

2. Close your eyes; you may prepare yourself by doing the abdominal-breathing exercise.

3. Let your eyes roll upward and inward a bit so that you focus on the spot on your forehead between your eyes, tongue resting behind your upper teeth, and all muscles as relaxed as possible. Smile inwardly in order to very subtly raise the corners of your mouth. As you repeat the focus word(s) silently, thoughts will enter your head. When you catch yourself on a random thought chase, be grateful to your "observer self" and then let the seductiveness of your mental chatter recede. It is normal—no matter how many years of practice—for the mind to be caught chasing its own tail. Smile inwardly and let the thoughts drift by as you breathe deeply and rhythmically.

4. You can time your words or phrases with your breath, keeping the inhalation broad, deep, and easy and the exhalation silent and effortless.

5. You can easily lose track of time in deep relaxation, so you may need to set a timer or stopwatch if you don't have unlimited time.

6. Remain seated for a minute or two with your eyes closed and then open them. Slowly begin to move your body, and ease yourself back into the world.

THE A-Z GUIDE

As simple as it sounds, some people cannot simply sit still "and do nothing." So if you're the kind of person who usually buzzes around, doing twelve things at once, don't be surprised if you can't sit quietly or if your mind wanders madly. If you have a flood of thoughts and your mind just won't quiet down, don't worry. Keep with it, and don't be too harsh on yourself if you feel you aren't "doing it." If you sit every day and just quietly let the thoughts pass without trying to stop them, and instead drift back to the mantra, word, or prayer, eventually the brain wave patterns begin to change. Deep physiological rest will occur and you will be meditating.

The meditation session itself is the goal; even if you think you're not doing it "right," you'll soon notice that you feel more peaceful and will feel relief from your symptoms. The more you practice, the more adept you'll get and the better you'll feel. Aim to meditate once a day, twice if possible. The best times are sunrise and sunset because, according to Robert Svoboda, Ayurvedic scholar and teacher, those are the times when both your nostrils are equally active, so you achieve a more complete, balanced meditation.

Mindfulness

This is another form of meditation that you do as you go about your daily life. It's a kind of "walking meditation" that brings your awareness to the moment, as opposed to the sitting-type meditation described earlier. Vata types tend to be quick and light in their thoughts, but when out of balance, thoughts turn chaotic. They are advised to meditate on their thinking process and watch their thoughts go by so that they become conscious of their pattern. It's characteristic of pittas to be discriminating; this is a gift, but they can get caught up in a web of being overly judgmental and so are advised to meditate on their judgments. Kapha's strength lies in its slow, steady, thought process. But when out of balance, thinking can become stuck and stagnant, so they are advised to be mindful of their thoughts and ask whether they are obsessing about the same thought again and again. By watching your thoughts, you stimulate thought, and can jog yourself out of stagnation.

AYURVEDA

YOGA

Yoga in Sanskrit means "union" and derives from the Hindu religion. It can be a spiritual practice that incorporates meditation and other mental exercises. A yoga session combined with mindful breathing can be a "moving meditation." There are many schools of yoga, but hatha yoga is the form most commonly practiced in Western countries, and classes and private lessons are available in health clubs, dance centers, yoga centers, and community centers. This form emphasizes physical postures called asanas and integrates them with breathing techniques.

Inactivity alone is responsible for much of the physical and mental deterioration we equate with illness, aging, and "feeling old." Practicing hatha yoga regularly not only relieves tension and pain in your joints and builds strength, flexibility, balance, and grace; it helps you reach a state of awareness, tranquility, and well-being. Practicing yoga regularly helps balance your nervous, endocrine, reproductive, digestive, and circulatory systems. Yoga knows no age limit—you're never too young or too old, and adherents age seventy and over remain astoundingly strong and limber.

The calmness achieved during the practice carries over into the rest of your life. Yoga students and teachers tend to look and act younger than their chronological years, and new students of the practice say they feel more energetic after only a few weeks' time. Although it can be strenuous, yoga is highly adaptable to your abilities and is suitable for people of all ages. You can learn yoga from books and videotapes, but it's best to participate in yoga classes (or get individual instruction), especially if you're new to the practice.

The basic yoga routine described on the next few pages is called the Sun Salutation. It is a full-body exercise that works on all the major muscle groups and joints and massages the internal organs. It should be performed joyously by everyone every day. We will be recommending additional specific yoga postures in the A–Z section.

THE A-Z GUIDE

Yoga is best performed on an empty stomach, in bare feet, while wearing loose or stretchy clothing, on a nonskid surface. There are special yoga "sticky mats" you can buy to prevent slipping and give you the most out of your practice. Breathing is an integral part of yoga because it is thought that prana, the vital life force, enters the body with each breath. As you practice yoga, coordinate your breathing with the movements: inhale during movements that stretch the spine and open the body; exhale during movements that involve bending or folding of the spine or limbs. Imagine that each breath is an extension of the pose, and keep your movements fluid and precise as you work to open up and extend your entire spine. Be conscious of your hands and feet as the foundation of each pose; imagine they are lotus blossoms, and spread your fingers and toes as if they were lotus petals.

We recommend that you perform the entire Sun Salutation sequence twelve times each morning. Begin slowly, with fewer repetitions, if you are new to yoga or physical activity. Gradually build up to twelve sequences, and rest when you need to, preferably in the Child's Pose. Vata types should continue to do these movements slowly, pittas should move at a moderate pace, and kaphas should aim to do them rapidly. As with any exercise program check with your doctor before beginning yoga.

Sun Salutation

When you have completed the sequence, rest in the Child's Pose until your breathing comes back to normal. You may also use this position to rest between sets if you need to. Then lie on your back, legs extended, arms at a 45-degree angle, and relax with your eyes closed for a few minutes.

AYURVEDA

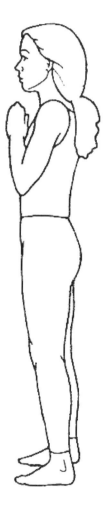

Sun Salutation Pose. Stand tall, feet hip-width apart and parallel. Place your palms together, prayer position, mid-chest. Take a few moments to become centered and focused.

THE A-Z GUIDE

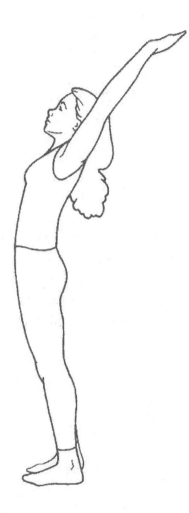

Raised-Arms Pose. Inhale as you stretch and sweep your arms out to the side and then overhead. Open your spine long, stretching your breastbone to the sky. You may arch your upper back slightly, but avoid arching the lower back or raising the shoulders.

AYURVEDA

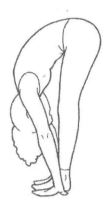

Hand-to-Foot Pose. Exhale as you bend over from the hips, sweeping your arms out to the side and placing your palms flat on the floor, one on each side of your feet. Ideally your knees should be straight but not locked; you may need to bend them at first to get your palms flat to the floor.

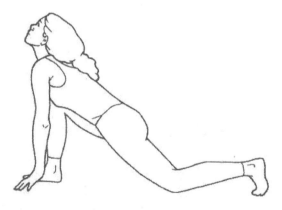

Lunge Pose. Inhale as you extend your left leg back in a lunge position. Position your right leg so that it makes a right angle, your calf perpendicular to the floor and your foot flat. It is preferable to keep your back leg straight and strong; you may drop the knee to the ground if you are a beginner. Remember to keep lengthening your spine and avoid hunching your shoulders or squeezing your neck.

THE A-Z GUIDE

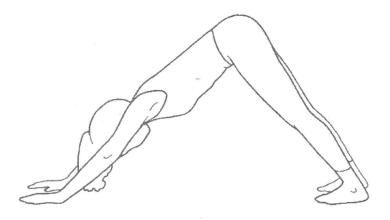

Downward Dog Pose. Exhale, bringing your right leg back to meet the left leg, feet hip-width apart. Lift your sitting bone up to the sky while you press down with your hands and feet, stretching your entire spine, shoulders, and backs of your legs. Keep your neck extended and relax your head.

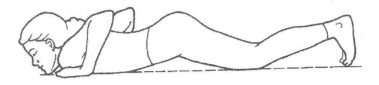

Eight-Limbs Pose. Hold your breath as you lower your knees to the ground and then bend your arms as you lower your chest and chin to the floor. Keep your toes curled under and your buttocks raised off the floor; the "eight limbs" are your feet, knees, hands, chest, and chin.

AYURVEDA

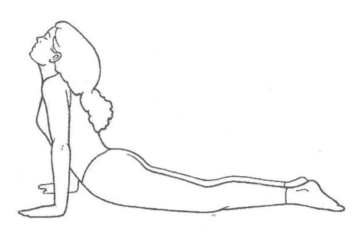

Cobra Pose. Inhale as you press down with your hands and begin to straighten your arms as you scoop your chest forward and up. Your elbows should remain close to your body and you should arch your lower back only as far as it can comfortably go. Move your breastbone up and out, and make sure to widen and drop your shoulders down away from your neck rather than scrunch your neck and shoulders together.

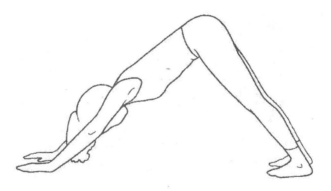

Downward Dog Pose. Exhale as you repeat this pose, trying to lengthen your spine even more as you press your hands and balls of your feet into the floor, stretching your heels down.

THE A-Z GUIDE

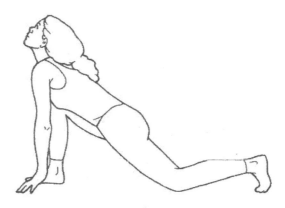

Lunge Pose. Inhale as you repeat this pose, bringing the right leg forward so that your foot is flat between your hands.

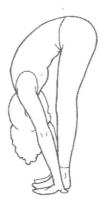

Hand-to-Foot Pose. Exhale as you step forward with the left foot and repeat this pose. Be careful not to round your upper back; the object is not to touch your head to your knee or to get your legs straight, but rather to extend and lengthen the spine out and over from the hips, not the waist.

AYURVEDA

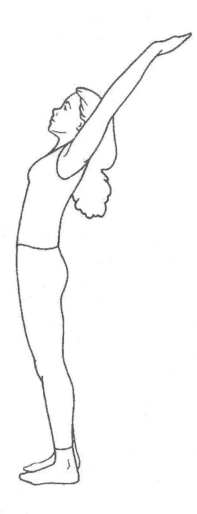

Raised-Arms Pose. Inhale deeply as you repeat this pose.

THE A-Z GUIDE

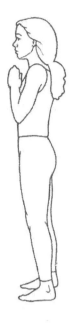

Sun Salutation Pose. Exhale as you bring your arms back to this pose. Take a few resting breaths before you repeat the set of twelve poses.

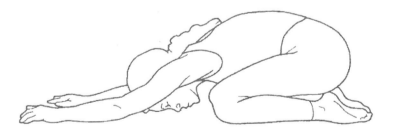

Child's Pose. Big toes touching, knees apart, sit back on your heels and bend at the hips, extending your arms on the floor in front of you.

CHAPTER FOUR

HEALING AYURVEDIC FOODS, HERBS, AND SPICES

Your kitchen cabinet is also your medicine cabinet because everyday foods, herbs, and spices can have medicinal as well as nutritional properties. What you ingest therefore can have a profound effect on your health. In this chapter we provide you with guidelines for specific foods you should emphasize or avoid, as well as herbs and spices you should keep on hand and use to gently balance the three doshas. Some items can be used every day, and for long periods of time. Others are appropriate for specific periods, such as short-course therapy to calm vata, the leading dosha, or increase agni, the digestive fire that is the cornerstone of Ayurvedic health. We also discuss the use of herbs and spices that are meant to be used for particular conditions, as recommended in the A–Z section. Many therapeutic herbs and spices are familiar inhabitants of your kitchen cabinet, others may be known to you as herbal remedies, and still others are unique to Ayurveda.

We begin with lists of everyday foods that the three individual doshas should emphasize, eat in moderation, or avoid. We then discuss the ways

THE A-Z GUIDE

Ayurveda uses herbs and spices in everyday cooking and in teas. Next you'll learn about herbs and spices that are more potent and concentrated; they are useful as medicines for specific complaints, such as those listed in the A–Z section. Finally, there are several recipes using combinations of small amounts of foods, herbs, and spices that Ayurveda considers to be therapeutic. Along with spice therapy, discussed in Chapter 5, the information in this chapter should open up a whole new world of taste to you. Remember to give yourself time to adjust to these new tastes in your life. Often when things don't taste good, it's because you've become habituated to a limited palate. Introducing all six tastes, in proportions appropriate for your dosha, restores your true metabolic alignment.

Eating the correct foods and herbs for your constitution can ease many problems, from indigestion to headache to fatigue. It can even cause excess pounds to disappear without your counting calories or depriving yourself. One patient says, "Since I began the Ayurvedic herbs three months ago, I released nineteen pounds and was no longer bothered with indigestion." Another patient attests:

"I had an amazing experience following the kapha diet. After sixteen years of battling overweight, I was able to feel more connected in just a few days. I went from feeling very bloated, thick, and heavy, to feeling just slightly bloated and very light. As time passed, I felt as if my inner swamp was draining, my digestive system was balancing itself, and my energy was becoming more even."

THE SIX TASTES

Foods contain packets of intelligence, or information, some of which are analyzed by our ability to taste. Herbs and spices are also potent food sources of these tastes, and therefore have become an important tool for stabilizing the doshas. Here's how the six tastes—sweet, sour, salty, bitter, pungent, and astringent—affect the doshas:

AYURVEDA

	VATA	PITTA	KAPHA
Stabilized by	Sweet,* Sour, Salty	Sweet,* Bitter, Astringent	Pungent, Bitter, Astringent
Aggravated by:	Bitter, Astringent, Pungent	Sour, Pungent, Salty	Sweet* Salty, Sour

COMMON EXAMPLES

Sweet: sugar*, milk, butter, rice, honey, bread

Sour: yogurt, lemon, cheese

Salty: salt, seaweed, soy sauce, pickles

Pungent: spicy foods, pepper, ginger, cumin

Bitter: spinach, other green leafy vegetables

Astringent: beans, pomegranate

*Refined white sugar is to be avoided by all the doshas; Sucanat, a new product made from the juice of organic sugar cane, is acceptable.

THE A-Z GUIDE

THE SIX QUALITIES

In addition to the six tastes, foods which are characterized according to six other qualities, which also affect the doshas and so must be taken into consideration. Generally doshas are aggravated by foods that have the same qualities as the dosha and are stabilized by those that have the opposite qualities:

	VATA	PITTA	KAPHA
Stabilized by	Heavy, Oily, Hot	Heavy, Oily, Cold	Light, Dry, Hot
Aggravated by	Light, Dry, Cold	Light, Dry, Hot	Heavy, Oily, Cold

Common Examples

Heavy: cheese, yogurt, wheat products, brown rice, red meat, sesame oil Light: barley, corn, spinach, apples, mung beans, basmati rice, chicken, sunflower oil

Oily: dairy products, fatty foods, oils, most nuts, eggs

Dry/drying: barley, corn, potatoes, beans, millet, pears

Hot/heating: heated food and drinks, sesame oil, meat, onions, eggs Cold/cooling: refrigerated or iced food and drink, milk, sunflower oil, coconut, wheat

AYURVEDA

FOOD GUIDELINES

Many things besides foods affect the doshas, including seasonal changes. For example during the vata season (late fall through winter), vata tends to be excessive in everyone, so Ayurveda recommends that during this time you eat foods that stabilize vata. Usually foods that come into season in your local region are the foods that tend to subdue the appropriate dosha. Generally therefore everyone should eat a variety of foods, but eat vata foods during the vata season, pitta foods during the pitta season, and kapha foods during the kapha season. Within the seasonal category there is a subset of foods that are most desirable; again using vata as an example, these would be seasonal foods that are sweet, salty, or sour, and that are heavy and oily, and that are eaten cooked and warm. If you are two-doshic (approximately equal amounts of two doshas), you can choose from both food groups when you are in balance. For example a pitta-vata can eat from both the pitta and the vata food lists.

Vata Foods

Use these guidelines for eating if . . .

- It is the vata season (late autumn through winter)
- Your prakruti is predominantly vata
- Your vata is aggravated

GENERAL PRINCIPLES

Eat and drink primarily foods that stabilize vata: warm foods and beverages, oily foods, foods that taste predominantly sweet, sour, or salty. Avoid foods that aggravate vata: light, dry foods, cold foods and drinks, and foods that taste predominantly pungent (spicy hot), bitter, or astringent. Eat regular meals and avoid skipping meals or fasting.

THE A-Z GUIDE

VEGETABLES

Emphasize avocados, sweet potatoes, parsley, cilantro, beets, seaweed, and chilies. Eat in moderation: peas, green beans, corn, artichokes, squash, turnips, okra, watercress, cauliflower, cucumbers, asparagus, celery, chard, spinach, mustard greens, and radishes. Avoid raw vegetables; eat small amounts of the following, but only if cooked: white potatoes, brussels sprouts, broccoli, cabbage, zucchini, onions. You may eat mung beans, tofu, kidney beans, lima beans, and chickpeas in moderation, but avoid pinto beans, lentils, split peas, and soybeans.

FRUITS

Emphasize lemons, limes, grapefruit, grapes, prunes, strawberries, raspberries, cherries, pineapples, dates, figs, mangoes, papayas. In moderation you may eat pears, bananas, oranges, peaches, apples (cooked), pomegranates, apricots, plums, and persimmons. Avoid cranberries, melons, and other dried fruits.

GRAINS

Emphasize rice, wheat, oats, and couscous. Eat moderate amounts of barley, corn, millet, buckwheat, rye, and quinoa.

NUTS, SEEDS, AND OILS

All nuts and oils are acceptable, but eat sunflower seeds, coconuts, and pumpkin seeds in moderation.

ANIMAL FOODS (NONVEGETARIANS)

All dairy products (except ice cream), eggs, fish, and shellfish may be eaten. Eat cheese, chicken, turkey, lamb, and beef in moderation; avoid pork.

AYURVEDA

SWEETENERS

Date sugar and fructose, barley malt, rice syrup, raw unrefined sugar; use Sucanat, fruit sugar, and honey in moderation; avoid white sugar.

Pitta Foods

Use these guidelines for eating if ...

- It is the pitta season (late spring through early autumn)
- Your prakruti is predominantly pitta
- Your pitta is aggravated

GENERAL PRINCIPLES

Eat and drink primarily foods that stabilize pitta: cool foods and drinks, and foods that taste predominantly sweet, bitter, and astringent. Reduce foods that increase your natural heat, such as foods that are predominantly pungent (spicy), sour, or salty.

VEGETABLES

Emphasize asparagus, pumpkin, cucumber, broccoli, cauliflower, avocado, celery, lettuce, zucchini, okra, green beans, mushrooms, alfalfa sprouts, cilantro, sunflower sprouts, brussels sprouts, cabbage, peas, adzuki beans, mung beans, lima beans, and tofu. Eat in moderation bell peppers, parsley, squash, corn, carrots, cooked onions, chard, spinach, beets, sweet potatoes, turnips, radishes, seaweed, watercress, split peas, soy, kidney beans, chickpeas, lentils.

FRUITS

Emphasize apples, cranberries, prunes, grapes, cherries, melons, coconut, pineapples, plums, mango, pears, and pomegranates. Reduce

THE A-Z GUIDE

raspberries, oranges, plums, mangoes, bananas, lemons, limes, papayas, persimmons. Avoid grapefruits.

GRAINS

Emphasize wheat, oats, barley, white rice, couscous, and quinoa. Eat moderate amounts of millet, brown rice, corn, lye, buckwheat.

NUTS, SEEDS, AND OILS

Emphasize sunflower seeds, coconut, ghee, butter, coconut oil; use in moderation pumpkin seeds, pine nuts, sesame seeds, peanuts, and olive, soy, sunflower, safflower, corn oils. Avoid cashews, walnuts, almonds, pecans, filberts, and sesame, almond, and peanut oil.

ANIMAL FOODS (NONVEGETARIANS)

Emphasize cream, milk, cottage cheese and cheese; use in moderation kefir, chicken, turkey, egg white, fish. Avoid sour cream, yogurt, buttermilk, ice cream, lamb, shellfish, pork, beef, and eggs.

SWEETENERS

Maple syrup, fructose, rice syrup, barley malt, raw unrefined sugar; use Sucanat, molasses, and honey in moderation; avoid white sugar.

Kapha Foods

Use these guidelines for eating if . . .

- It is the kapha season (early spring through early summer)
- Your prakruti is predominantly kapha
- Your kapha is aggravated

AYURVEDA

GENERAL PRINCIPLES

Your diet should consist primarily of foods and beverages that stabilize kapha and are stimulating: choose foods that are light, dry, and warm and that taste primarily pungent (spicy), bitter, or astringent. Avoid overeating and foods and beverages that aggravate kapha, such as those that are oily, cold, or predominantly sweet, sour, or salty.

VEGETABLES

Emphasize asparagus, cilantro, mushrooms, broccoli, cabbage, lettuce, alfalfa sprouts, mustard greens, chard, turnips, watercress, radishes, beets, carrots, pumpkin, celery, peas, green beans, chilies, lentils, lima and soybeans. Eat moderate amounts of parsley, cauliflower, spinach, okra, squash, corn, seaweeds, chickpeas, split peas, tofu, and kidney and mung beans. Avoid cucumbers, avocado, and sweet potatoes.

FRUITS

Emphasize apples, cranberries, and dried fruits. Eat grapefruits, pomegranates, prunes, lemons, limes, and papayas in moderation. Avoid grapes, bananas, pineapples, oranges, pears, melons, plums, cherries, strawberries, mangoes, dates, and figs.

GRAINS

Emphasize quinoa and barley; eat moderate amounts of corn, millet, buckwheat, rye, and basmati rice. Avoid couscous, oats, brown or white rice, and wheat.

NUTS, SEEDS, AND OILS

Emphasize safflower, sunflower, and mustard oils; eat small quantities of coconut, and pumpkin, sunflower, and sesame seeds, ghee, and corn, peanut, and soy oils. Avoid walnuts, cashews, almonds, pine nuts,

THE A-Z GUIDE

filberts, pecans, Brazil nuts and their oils, as well as butter, sesame, olive, and avocado oils.

ANIMAL FOODS (NONVEGETARIANS)

Use moderate amounts of buttermilk, goat milk, and kefir, and turkey and chicken; avoid all other animal and daily products.

SWEETENERS

Use only honey, fruit-juice concentrates, and Sucanat in moderation.

HERBS AND SPICES

Ayurveda has its own unique view of herbs and spices and how they work. Herbs are thought of, first of all, as a kind of concentrated food. In Ayurveda herbs and spices are regularly consumed in cooked foods and as flavorful teas. Thus you can easily integrate them into your life. Based on the results of the self-assessments in Chapter 2, you can use herbs on a daily basis to help balance your doshas, and energize, sustain, and strengthen vitality, enliven the mind, rejuvenate the tissues, and strengthen the immune system. Second, certain herbs and spices are stronger and have more pronounced effects on the mind-body; these are used medicinally for short periods of time to treat specific conditions, as you'll see in the A-Z section.

Buying and Using Herbs and Spices

Although herbs affect the body through several discrete mechanisms— they contain vitamins, minerals, hormones, and chemicals that act as stimulants and relaxants, and so on—Ayurveda traditionally classifies them according to their taste, which in turn becomes a guide to their use. This is why Ayurveda doesn't employ herbal tinctures, whose alcohol base would influence the taste; and generally doesn't use tablets or capsules either, because taking herbs in this form would bypass the taste-buds and reduce the herbs' effectiveness.

AYURVEDA

Most herbs and spices are used in powdered form for both cooking and medicinal purposes. Some herbs and spices may be sold as seeds or pods that you can grind or crush with a mortar and pestle; fresh ginger is a commonly used herb that you grate before use. You can buy the herbs we recommend for cooking and teas at most health food stores, farmers' markets, and many food markets. Many of the medicinal herbs are not as readily available; you will find them at Indian grocery stores and from the mail-order sources listed in Appendix B. Make sure your herbs are fresh when you buy them, and store them in a dark dry place for up to one year (mark the expiration date on the container).

COOKING WITH HERBS AND SPICES

Herbs and spices add flavor while balancing the doshas. Experiment with the herbs and spices listed below, or use one of the Ayurvedic cookbooks (see Appendix D), which will teach you how to prepare delicious, flavorful foods that taste good and are good for you. To calm vata, emphasize sweet, sour, and salty herbs, spices, and flavorings, such as fresh ginger, fennel, oregano, sage, tarragon, thyme, cinnamon, basil, cardamom, coriander, and cumin.

To cool pitta, emphasize herbs and spices that are sweet, bitter, and astringent, such as fresh cilantro, fresh ginger, cumin, coriander, fennel, chamomile, turmeric, mint, cinnamon, cardamom, and nutmeg.

To stimulate kapha, emphasize herbs and spices that are pungent, bitter, and astringent, such as black pepper, cayenne, garlic, mustard, fresh ginger, cinnamon, cloves, cardamom, turmeric, coriander, fresh cilantro, and cumin.

To reduce gas from beans, broccoli, brussels sprouts, cabbage, onions, and so forth, add a combination of turmeric, cumin, coriander, fennel, cinnamon, or cayenne pepper. This is especially helpful for vata types.

THE A-Z GUIDE

To make milk more digestible, use cardamom, cinnamon, and ginger.

Spiced herbal teas are a gentle yet effective way to use herbs and spices every day. "Yogi tea," available at some health food stores, is an all-purpose blend beneficial for all doshas. There are also commercially available herbal blends labeled vata-pacifying, pitta-pacifying, or kapha-pacifying, designed for specific doshas. And there are also formulas designed to treat specific symptoms, such as indigestion, fatigue, insomnia, and colds, available as tea bags. Keep these teas on hand and use them regularly to restore or maintain balance. Alternatively you can make your own yogi, vata, pitta, and kapha teas using the recipes provided.

MEDICINAL HERBS AND SPICES

Herbs have been called part of "nature's pharmacy." Although their action can in some ways be similar to modern drugs, herbal remedies are generally gentler and safer. Many of the drugs used in conventional medicine are derived from herbs, but rather than isolating the "active agent," herbalism uses the whole plant or whole parts of the plant, such as the leaves, the flowers, or the roots. Frequently plants contain constituents that work together synergistically. Sometimes using the whole plant helps decrease the side effects that may occur when using isolated components. When you turn to the A–Z section, you will see that many herbs and spices are recommended, usually in combination, to treat specific conditions. In contrast to herbs used in everyday cooking, medicinal herbs are more powerful and are usually prescribed for only a short period of time.

To make the formulas we suggest, buy individual herbs and spices and combine them as needed, or mix a bigger batch ahead of time and store in a jar so that you can take what you need per dose. Such combinations are generally mixed with warm water or milk, or with honey. Herbs may also be cooked in ghee (clarified butter, see recipe). These are known as medicated ghees and are especially useful because we live in a world of high technology and are bombarded with electromagnetic fields. These

AYURVEDA

medicated ghees provide lubrication and a vehicle for the herbs to better penetrate the tissues and therefore be more effective.

There are herbal-formula tablets and capsules that are commercially available for specific conditions and syndromes, but as mentioned earlier, these are less preferable than powdered herbs that you mix with a liquid or ghee and drink or eat and thus expose to your taste buds. For example the Maharishi Ayurveda Company makes Ayurvedic formulas designed to act as antioxidants, to aid digestion, to relieve insomnia and nervousness, to improve mental clarity, and for women at midlife that help nourish and balance the hormones. In recent studies two of these compounds (they go by the names MAK 4 and MAK 5) have been found to be nontoxic while they enhance the immune system; reduce platelet aggregation (clumping), a risk factor in heart disease; reduce the incidence of breast cancer in rats by up to 88 percent; cause up to 60 percent of tumors to regress; and prevent the spread of experimentally induced lung cancer in up to 66 percent of animals tested. They have also been found to contain antioxidants, which suggests they may be useful in reducing cell damage and illness caused by free radicals—molecules associated with tissue damage associated with aging and dozens of degenerative diseases. A clinical study conducted in India found that cancer patients who received these formulas along with chemotherapy experienced fewer toxic side effects.

Commercially prepared capsules or tablets are expensive, but may be preferable if you simply can't get used to the taste of particular herbs, or in the case of a substance such as cayenne pepper, which needs to be taken in capsule form to insulate you from the burning sensation. You can make your own capsules by filling "00" gelatin capsules.

There are many medicinal compounds used in Ayurveda; some of the most commonly recommended formulas include the following:

Triphala, a traditional herbal cleansing compound that is used as an all-around tonic. It helps balance all three doshas and is composed of three fruits in dried, powdered form, hence the name, tri-phala. The three

THE A-Z GUIDE

fruits are amalaki (pitta-cooling and balancing), haritaki (vatawarming and balancing), and bibhitaki (kapha-stimulating and balancing). Triphala is the mainstay in treating and preventing many conditions; unlike other Ayurvedic herbal formulas, triphala may be taken for several months. Triphala is generally taken mixed with warm water and consumed as a tea upon arising or before bedtime. Take one-half to one full teaspoon daily, alone or along with other herbal remedies suggested in this chapter and under the A—Z listings of common conditions. (See Appendix B for suppliers.)

Trikatu is another mainstay and consists of black pepper, long pepper, and dried ginger; its uses include the treatment of indigestion, cough, low agni, and weak digestive fire.

Guggula compounds come in several types, each made with the resin of guggul, a relative of myrrh. They are used primarily to treat nervous system disorders. Guggula may also be combined with yogarash, ginger, and triphala to produce a purification compound.

Ashwagandha (winter cherry) is often combined with licorice and turmeric and used as a general male toner.

Shatavari is often combined with licorice and turmeric for a female toner.

RECIPES FOR AYURVEDIC HEALTH

Certain combinations of foods, herbs, and spices can be taken on a regular basis as gentle medicines to help restore your mind-body's natural balance. What follows is a selection of specific recipes for delicious teas, soups, and meals that you can incorporate into your daily menus as part of your self-healing.

AYURVEDA

Spiced Herbal Teas

Make a pot of tea in the morning; have one cup at breakfast, instead of coffee, black tea, or your usual caffeine and/or sugar-laden beverage. Drink the rest throughout the day (take some in a thermos to work). You can experiment with the proportions of herbs and spices to get a blend that most pleases your palate; just aim to use one teaspoon total per brewed cup of tea.

YOGI TEA

This is a tri-doshic tea, good for general balancing of all three doshas. Boil 8 cups water in a stainless steel saucepan. Add:

    2 teaspoons fresh grated ginger
    4 whole cardamom seeds, slightly crushed
    1 whole cinnamon stick, slightly crushed 8 whole cloves

Boil for 20 minutes. Strain and drink warm or cooled to room temperature, and add sweetener and milk if desired. •

VATA-STABILIZING TEA

This tea calms vata, which goes out of balance by becoming aggravated. Boil 4 cups water in a stainless steel saucepan. Reduce heat and stir in

    2 teaspoons fresh grated ginger
    1 teaspoon whole cardamom seeds, slightly crushed
    2 whole cinnamon sticks, slightly crushed
    1/8 teaspoon saffron
    1 teaspoon dried orange peel (optional)

Let simmer, covered, for 10 minutes. Remove from heat and let steep 5 more minutes. To serve, strain and add fresh boiled milk and honey, if desired. This makes about 3 1/2 cups of tea. You may reheat it or drink it at room temperature.

THE A-Z GUIDE

PITTA-STABILIZING TEA

Chamomile or mint teas are simple, easy teas to brew for soothing pitta. The following combination more forcefully cools and strengthens pitta, which goes out of balance by becoming overheated. Boil 4 cups water in a stainless steel saucepan. Remove pan from heat and stir in:

    2 teaspoons fresh grated ginger
    1 teaspoon whole cardamom seeds, slightly crushed
    1 1/2 teaspoon spearmint or other mint
    2 whole cinnamon sticks, slightly crushed
    1/8 teaspoon fennel seeds (optional)

Cover the tea and let steep for at least 10 minutes. To serve, strain, squeezing out as much of the liquid as you can; add maple syrup if desired. This makes about 3 1/2 cups of strong tea; dilute with 2 cups water if it seems too strong for you. Sip hot or at room temperature as desired.

KAPHA-STABILIZING TEA

This stimulating beverage serves to invigorate kapha mentally and physically, which tends to become more sluggish when out of balance. Boil 4 cups water in a stainless steel saucepan. Reduce heat and stir in:

    1 teaspoon whole cardamon seeds, slightly crushed 1 teaspoon whole cloves
    1/8 teaspoon black pepper
    1 tablespoon peeled and chopped fresh ginger 1 teaspoon dried gotu kola (optional)

Let simmer, covered, for at least 10 minutes. To serve, strain and add honey to sweeten if desired. This makes about 3-1/2 cups.

AYURVEDA

Ghee

Ayurveda considers ghee, or clarified butter, to be the most important lubricant you can ingest. One of our teachers compared it with oil for your engine; a small amount goes a long way and is essential for the life of your car. The same is true of ghee and its relationship to your body. Ghee helps create ojas, improve sexual vitality, strengthen your nervous system, and build muscle. Ghee is used for cooking, particularly for sautéing vegetables; as a flavoring for vegetables or grains and cereals; and as an ingredient in herbal medicines that allows the herbs to penetrate deep into the tissues. To make ghee:

1. Put one pound of unsalted organic butter in a stainless steel or heat-proof glass pan and place over medium heat.

2. Allow to melt and come to a boil; skim off the foam that forms on top. Lower the heat and simmer until the ghee turns deep golden brown, but do not burn it.

3. Remove from heat, let cool, and strain into a storage jar. Store in your refrigerator, where it will keep in definitely. Ghee will last up to two months without refrigeration.

Copper Water

This is an inexpensive, simple, and traditional Ayurvedic method to ingest copper, a trace metal that is required for many physiological processes. In some locales where the plumbing consists of copper pipes, people get plenty of copper, but in most locales the soil is so depleted of copper that some source other than food or water is needed. Some advise drinking copper water every day upon arising, whereas others prefer to use it as a specific treatment in certain instances, as for example in a person who is at high risk for cardiovascular problems. Copper water is used in a few of the remedies in the A–Z section. To make copper water, pour water into a copper cup; cover with a glass lid and let sit overnight.

THE A-Z GUIDE

Ten-Day Ginger Treatment

Ginger has many uses in Ayurveda, depending on the dosage and how you take it. In this traditional use it improves agni, or the digestive fire, and can be used by anyone. Mix together 8 teaspoons each of grated fresh ginger, brown sugar or succanat, and melted ghee (see ghee recipe). Store in your refrigerator, and each morning before breakfast take the amount listed below. This remedy is surprisingly delicious, and the gingery, buttery, sugary taste stays with you all day. (Note: Vegans may substitute grapeseed oil for ghee.)

Day 1:   1/2 teaspoon
Day 2:   1 teaspoon
Day 3:   1 1/2 teaspoon
Day 4:   2 teaspoons
Day 5:   2 1/2 teaspoons
Day 6:   2 1/2 teaspoons
Day 7:   2 teaspoons
Day 8:   1 1/2 teaspoons
Day 9:   1 teaspoon
Day 10: 1/2 teaspoon

Juice-and-Soup Fast

In order to help reduce ama accumulation, Ayurveda recommends that you do this purification technique once a week to stabilize kapha and once every two weeks to stabilize vata or pitta. Everyone should do this fast for four to five days during the transition between the seasons. Eat four to six servings of soup per day. Drink at least sixteen ounces divided throughout the day.

AYURVEDA

SOUP (makes 1 to 2 servings):

    3 cups water
    1 handful mung dahl (yellow lentils, available at Indian food stores)
    1 medium broccoli spear
    3 medium celery stalks cut up
    2 medium zucchini squashes cut up
    2 medium carrots, cut up
    2 leaves each collard greens, kale, and chard
    A few sprigs parsley
    1 teaspoon sea salt

Wash mung dahl, bring to a boil in the water, and add vegetables and salt. Reduce heat to low and cook, covered, at least 1/2 hour, or until dahl is soft.

Next sauté over low heat:

    1 tablespoon ghee
    1 teaspoon whole black mustard seeds 1 teaspoon whole cumin seeds
    1 teaspoon fenugreek seeds

When seeds begin to pop, add:

    1 teaspoon fresh grated ginger
    1 1/2 teaspoons freshly ground coriander seeds
    1/2 teaspoon turmeric
    1/4 teaspoon ground black pepper

Place the ghee mixture into a blender; add 1 cup cooked soup. Blend for a few seconds, add the rest of the soup, and blend again.

JUICES

Vegetable juices: wheat grass, beets, carrots, kale, parsley

Fruit juices are to be taken alone.

Kicharee

Kicharee is a medicinal meal and was used traditionally to bring very sick people back to health. You may eat this special dish whenever you are recovering from an illness.

 1/4 cup split mung dahl (yellow lentils)
 1/2 cup basmati rice
 2 tablespoons ghee or sunflower oil
 1/4 teaspoon cumin seeds
 3 bay leaves
 1 teaspoon coriander 1 teaspoon oregano 1/2 teaspoon turmeric
 4 to 6 cups water
 1/2 teaspoon salt
 1 stick kombu
 1 teaspoon fresh grated ginger
 3 cups diced fresh vegetables such as carrots, zucchini, and summer squash

Wash the beans and rice until the water runs clear. Warm the ghee in a medium saucepan; add the cumin, bay leaves, coriander, and oregano. Brown slightly until their aroma is released. Stir in turmeric, rice, and dahl. Add water, salt, Kombu, and ginger. Simmer, covered, over medium heat for about 1 hour, or until the beans and rice are soft. Add vegetables and cook 10 to 15 minutes more, or until tender.

AYURVEDA

PRECAUTIONS FOR TAKING HERBS

- If you are presently taking medications, or are under medical treatment for a specific medical condition, it is essential to consult your health professional before administering Ayurvedic medicines. Some herbs should be avoided or used under the guidance of a professional if you have a chronic illness or a diagnosed medical problem; for example licorice contains plant hormones that may stimulate uterine bleeding and may also stimulate the growth of breast and uterine tissue, which is a concern for women who have a history of estrogen-sensitive cancers or a high risk for them.

- Do not combine herbs with prescription or over-the-counter medications unless you are under professional supervision; some herbs may contain similar substances and could result in an overdose. If you have any questions or doubts, contact a knowledgeable herb specialist for advice.

- Remember to use caution when using herbs. In some people certain herbs may cause undesirable reactions. Begin with the lowest recommended dosage and gradually increase as needed. The most common symptoms of herb intolerance are nausea; vomiting, diarrhea, or allergic reactions; however, these are rare and extremely variable depending on both the herb and the individual. If you notice any questionable reaction, discontinue the herb(s) at once. If your reaction is severe, call your local Poison Control Center and go to the emergency room of the nearest hospital.

- Read the manufacturer's recommendations carefully and do not use any herbal product that does not supply detailed information on appropriate dosages. There have been reports of mislabeling of herbs, and quality and potency can vary depending on harvesting, handling, and storage. Therefore be sure to buy herbs only from the most reputable sources you can find.

CHAPTER FIVE

FIVE-SENSE THERAPY: KEEPING ALL THE DOORS OPEN

According to Ayurveda, the five senses are the doorways to our internal physiology. Your brain has ten billion nerve cells, and over one trillion different electrical circuits. Your five senses fill these circuits day and night with a ceaseless perseverance. But the brain is only one part of you. As Diane Ackerman writes in The Natural History of the Senses,

> Most people think of the mind as located in the head, but the latest findings in physiology suggest that the mind doesn't really dwell in the brain but travels the whole body on caravans of hormones and enzymes, busily making sense of the compound wonders we catalogue as touch, taste, smell, hearing, and vision.

Choosing the precise medicine for your one trillion circuits and 10 trillion cells can make the difference between inner serenity and inner chaos, between health and disease. This chapter discusses the underlying rationale for the five-sense therapy we use in our clinical practice to restore and maintain balance to the doshas. The simple practices suggested here are among the most pleasurable and effective in Ayurveda and include making use of fragrant essential oils, tasty spices, wondrous musical compositions, and special massage points.

In our clinic Ayurvedic therapy often begins with five-sense therapy because it is so easy and pleasurable for her patients to use—and because of its speedy effect. For example one patient says that "after Dr. Thomas had me use light, sound, and aromatherapy, I immediately felt better: more relaxed, balanced, and energetic." The five-sense therapies are

AYURVEDA

even more effective if you use them in conjunction with other fundamental Ayurvedic practices, as this patient discovered: "Five days after I began light therapy, raga music, vata aromatherapy, using herbal oil for daily self-massage, and following the vata-stabilizing diet, I could feel the energetic shift happening."

You, too, can use these easy at-home techniques as adjuncts to the basic prevention, rejuvenation, and longevity practices taught in Chapter 3 and the kitchen medicines described in Chapter 4. In addition to general balancing, the five-sense therapies are also useful for treating specific conditions, as recommended in the A–Z section. Remember, while a single-sense therapy used alone is often helpful and provides symptom relief, using all five together will penetrate more completely to the underlying cause of the condition.

USING ALL FIVE SENSES

Before focusing on specific sense therapies, try this exercise to enhance your awareness of what you take in through your senses. Visit a place in nature. Close your eyes and be silent for five minutes, recording in your mind everything you hear, smell and feel. Open your eyes and do the same with what you see. You may want to write down your observations as well. Then perform the same exercise on a busy highway overpass, your workplace, a shopping mall, or the heart of a big-city downtown. When you compare how you felt in these various places, it should be clear to you why we recommend that you spend some time in nature every day. Choose a balcony, a garden, a park, a wilderness area—but to capture inner peace and connectedness with the earth, you need to see natural sights, hear natural sounds, smell natural aromas, and feel the wind caress your cheek and the grass beneath your feet.

While the practices outlined here have direct health benefits, they also prime your sense to absorb all forms of sensual pleasures. An excellent source of ideas, inspiration, and information on everyday ways to enrich

THE A-Z GUIDE

your life is a book called Healthy Pleasures by Robert Ornstein and David Sobel. In it the authors present the growing evidence that feeling good is good for you—pleasure is nature's way of guiding us to experiences that enhance health.

TASTE: SPICE THERAPY

Taste is of profound importance in the way Ayurveda understands the human mind-body. In Ayurveda each taste is an energetic bundle of information picked up by the tongue's taste buds. There are nine thousand taste buds, and when stimulated they trigger nerve impulses to special taste centers in the brain's cortex and thalamus. These tastes, called rasas, are recognized as sweet, sour, salty, bitter, pungent, or astringent. If you don't have all six tastes every day, your brain is being deprived of nourishing stimulation.

How Taste Affects the Doshas

- Sweet is composed of the elements of earth and water. It is the taste of pleasure; it makes us feel comforted and content, and that's why so many mothers instinctively try to pacify their babies with sweet treats. In Ayurveda the sweet taste in the form of food and spices is considered to be one of the most healing tools for any debilitating weakness. In Ayurveda sweet is most balancing for the young and old, and for vata and pitta; it aggravates kapha. Sweet refers to the taste of natural sugars in many fruits including peaches, sweet plums, grapes, melons, and oranges; vegetables such as sweet potatoes, carrots, and beets; milk, butter, and whole grains such as rice and wheat bread; and herbs and spices such as basil, licorice, and fennel. In your quest for sweet taste Ayurveda recommends that you avoid highly processed sweets such as candy bars, which also contain additives, food coloring, and preservatives.

AYURVEDA

- Salt is composed of water and fire and is found in table salt, rock salt, sea salt, and seaweeds. A basic unit of electricity, salt helps vata retain moisture; pitta and kapha types should use salt in moderation. Salt creates flexibility in the joints, increases digestive activity, and improves the taste of food. Too much salt causes wrinkles, thirst, skin disorders, and weakness.

- Sour, composed of earth and fire, creates a feeling of adventurousness. Close your eyes. See a tart, juicy yellow lemon. Imagine taking the lemon into your mouth—your teeth may tingle, your lips and eyes may squeeze shut and water, barely able to stand the zest. The sour taste is also found in other citrus fruits; pickles; miso (fermented soybean paste); vinegar; yogurt; cheese; and sour cream; and in herbs such as caraway, coriander, and cloves. It is good for the heart, digestion, and assimilation. It increases kapha and pitta and decreases vata; if you take in too much sour, you can become weak and giddy.

- Bitter is the taste composed of air and space. Most Americans are unfamiliar with the bitter taste, except in their coffee, which they usually modify with sweetener and cream. Yet bitterness is considered to be one of the most healing tastes for many kinds of imbalances in the mind-body. Bitter foods and herbs are drying and cooling and create lightness, and thus are balancing for kapha and pitta, but aggravating for vata. Too much bitter in the diet will cause dehydration. Rhubarb, bitter melon, and greens such as Romaine lettuce, spinach, and chard are bitter; as are fenugreek and turmeric.

- Pungent is composed of fire and air. It improves taste and digestion, provides heat and dryness, and stimulates stagnant emotional ama. The pungent taste balances kapha, which requires it in the diet; it should be used in small amounts by vatas, who are warmed but easily dried out by it. Pittas, with their natural heat, need very little, and people with pitta imbalances should avoid pungent foods altogether. Spicy and hot foods, such as onion, garlic, cayenne pepper, black pepper, mustard, and ginger, are pungent.

- Astringent, composed of air and earth, is probably the least familiar taste to the American mind and palate. Astringent foods and herbs squeeze out water; they are whatever makes your mouth pucker after eating them and include apples, cranberries, pomegranates, okra, beans, mace, parsley, saffron, and basil. Astringent taste is balancing for kaphas, who tend to have excess water, and pittas, but aggravating for vatas, who are dry already.

How to Use Spice Therapy

The foods, herbs, and spices recommended in Chapter 4 for general balancing are in part based on the unique effect each taste has on the doshas. Taste is also one of the determinants of Ayurvedic pharmacology and is the basis for its spice therapy. The simplest, least expensive way to incorporate spice therapy into your life is through the use of churnas. Churnas are combinations of powdered spices with all six tastes with either vata-, pitta-, or kapha-type spices predominating. To use, you simply sprinkle the mixture on your food at least once a day, just like salt and pepper.

You can use the following recipes to make your own churnas. Buy the herbs and spices individually (see Chapter 3 for information on buying and storing), combine, and keep in a handy shaker jar.

SUMMER CHURNA

Stabilizes pitta; use from summer to late fall. Combine 1 part each cinnamon, cardamom, licorice, poppy seed, turmeric, and sugar with 1/2 part nutmeg.

AYURVEDA

WINTER CHURNA

Stabilizes vata; use from late fall to late winter, depending on the severity of the climate you live in.

Combine 1 part each cinnamon, cumin, fennel, fenugreek, and ginger with 112 part each salt and pepper.

SPRING CHURNA

Stabilizes kapha; use from early spring to early summer.

Combine 1 part each cloves, dill, celery, ginger, cumin, tarragon, and pepper with 1 / 2 part garlic.

SMELL: AROMATHERAPY

The sense of smell is vastly underappreciated—it can give you early warning of a nearby fire, arouse your sexual interest or appetite for food, and elicit a surge of deep-seated memories. Without smell you couldn't distinguish the taste of an apple from that of an onion or potato: 80 percent of your ability to detect a flavor comes from fragrances. How can a mere sniff be so powerful?

Smell owes its potency to the fact that, unlike other senses, it is directly connected with the emotion-generating areas in the brain. When you inhale an aroma, its molecules stimulate two tiny membranes deep in your nose. They stimulate receptors that trigger an electric signal to the limbic system and the hypothalamus. These ancient parts of the brain activate, control, and integrate parts of the nervous system, endocrine system, and many body functions including heart rate, respiration, temperature, blood sugar levels, waking, sleeping, and sexual arousal. They are also the seat of your most basic emotions—such as pleasure, anger, sadness, and fear—and are involved in memory.

THE A-Z GUIDE

How Aromas Affect the Doshas

Aromatherapy, the use of specific essential aromatic oils, is an Ayurvedic treatment for correcting imbalances in the doshas. This therapy works by penetrating into the memory and breaking the pattern of imbalance that lives there. In this way aromatherapy heals the memory of trauma and disease, quickly, effortlessly, and pleasurably.

- Vata is calmed by warm, sweet, sour smells such as basil, orange, rose geranium, and clove. Vata tends to be fearful when out of balance, and aromatherapy cultivates positive vata emotions of joy and inventiveness.

- Pitta is balanced by sweet, cool aromas such as sandalwood, rose, mint, cinnamon, and jasmine. With aromatherapy pitta's irritability and anger are replaced with creativity and enthusiasm.

- Kapha responds to pungent aromas such as juniper, eucalyptus, camphor, clove, and marjoram. These fragrances stimulate kapha out of its cynicism and apathy and toward extroversion, sociability, and energy.

How to Use Aromatherapy

There are many ways you can easily and simply use the above combinations of aromatic essential oils to stabilize each dosha and its predominant emotions. You can place a few drops of the oils into a special ring made to be placed over a light bulb; this disperses the fragrance as long as the bulb is on. You can use a special diffuser, which uses candle power to heat water containing the oils. You can make a spray with a combination of the oil, water, and lecithin (to get the oil and water to mix). You can sprinkle the oil in your bath. Just before bed is ideal for aromatherapy, but anytime is appropriate.

AYURVEDA

Precautions: Never take essential oils internally. Also, be sure to dilute essential oils with a carrier oil before applying to the skin. The most commonly used carrier oil is sesame, which is particularly suited to vata types and vata disorders; coconut is preferred for pitta; and flaxseed or almond oil for kapha. The usual ratio is 10 drops essential oil per 4 ounces of carrier oil.

SIGHT: COLOR THERAPY

If you've ever seen natural sunlight pass through a prism, you've experienced with your own eyes how light is composed of all the colors of the rainbow. What you may not realize is that it is light that you see when you perceive a solid object. All objects absorb some of the light waves and reflect others. For example a red apple absorbs most of the blue and yellow light waves, but not the red ones. Your eye picks up the light waves that bounce off the object's surface and sends them to the brain, which interprets them for you as "red."

Light feeds the brain, particularly the area of the brain known as the hypothalamus. The hypothalamus regulates and controls the adrenals, pituitary, thymus, and entire endocrine system. We know that without proper exposure to light, disorders develop. For example the well-documented SAD (seasonal affective disorder) is a type of depression that is treated successfully with full-spectrum light therapy. Without light plants—indeed all forms of life on earth—would cease to exist. Sun-worshiping cultures recognize that the very source of life is the sun.

How Color and Light Affect the Doshas

The color messages sent by light waves affect the doshas and hence your health.

Vatas do best with yellow, orange, and white; small amounts of red, green, blue, and violet are also stabilizing. They should avoid black, gray, brown, and all dark colors.

THE A-Z GUIDE

Pittas do best with white, green, and blue; gray and brown may be used in small amounts. Pittas should avoid strong, bright colors such as red and black.

Kaphas do best with red, orange, and golden yellows; black, gray, and brown may be used in lesser amounts. Avoid white, pink, and pale green or blue.

In addition to these overall guidelines, certain colors have specific benefits; for example:

- Red builds blood, improves red blood cell production, improves circulation, and inspires the creative process.
- Yellow stimulates agni, increases assimilation, and raises consciousness.
- Orange fights bacteria, strengthens the immune system, and instills knowledge.
- Blue is cooling, enhances perception, and reduces pain.
- Green is calming, refreshing, and energizing.

How to Use Color and Light Therapy

The healthiest form of light is sunlight, or full-spectrum artificial light that mimics sunlight. In addition to being out in the sunshine for at least twenty minutes every day and introducing as much natural sunlight into your home and workplace as possible, you can emphasize certain specific colors in your surroundings (furnishings, wall and floor coverings, clothing, and so on) to help balance your doshas and support your health.

You can also use the following form of color-energized light therapy, which we refer to in the A–Z section in recommending specific color combinations. Here's how it works: Place a sheet of theatrical gel in the recommended color around a clear glass jar. Fill the jar with boiled

AYURVEDA

water and place it in a window that gets diffused sunlight. Leave the jar in the window during eight daylight hours. Every day drink up to four ounces of the water within two to three hours of taking the filter off the jar. You will need to change the gel periodically to keep the concentration of color strong.

HEARING: SOUND THERAPY

It's obvious that people respond to sound—a screaming siren affects you differently than a songbird, classical music has a different effect from that of jazz. Science has confirmed that music, an organized form of sound, can directly affect mood, brain waves, and body chemistry.

How Music Affects Health

Music plays a key role in the spiritual and religious' rituals of many cultures arid is often considered to be a healing salve. Western medicine and dentistry use music primarily to calm and relax patients, with such classical pieces as Bach's "Air on the G String," Pachelbel's Canon, Haydn's Cello Concerto in C, Debussy's "Claire de Lune," and Gregorian chants, as well as with nonclassical music. Music therapists also recognize that some people may require stimulating music to energize them toward better health.

Music has been found to enhance immune function; improve thinking ability; improve sleep; exercise, and work performance; help speed recovery from heart attacks and strokes; reduce side effects of chemotherapy; ease chronic pain; reduce the amount of anesthesia required during surgery; and reduce the amount of painkiller required during childbirth. And of course Musak in stores has been used for years to seduce people into buying their wares.

You may want to experiment with various musical compositions to see how they affect you. However, certain ragas, the traditional Hindu music, offer a much more sophisticated and finely tuned, yet universal, instrument for healing.

THE A-Z GUIDE

Raga in Sanskrit means "musical color." There are medicinal ragas, composed and played to heal the sick. The Ayurvedic approach to music therapy is based on the observation that different times of day have different vibratory qualities. The early morning, when the day is fresh and birds awaken and the dew is on the leaves, vibrates at a different frequency, for instance, from midday or the deep, dark velvet of late night.

Ayurveda uses music that is based on these changing rhythms of the day. In this form of music, ragas are created according to the following eight three-hour segments of the day:

7 to 10 A.M.: sunrise
10 A.M. to 1 P.M.: midmorning 1 to 4 P.M.: midday
4 to 7 P.M.: late afternoon 7 to 10 P.M.: sunset
10 P.M. to 1 A.M.: late evening 1 to 4 A.M.: midnight
4 to 7 A.M.: predawn

Of course these precise times vary with the seasons, but sunrise always marks the beginning of the first segment.

How to Use Raga Sound Music Therapy

Listening to the raga appropriate for the time of day is considered to be stabilizing for all three doshas. As with the other senses, your doshas react to sound vibrations, and thus you can use this music to balance them whenever they become out of sync with the rhythms of the day. The notes, rhythms, and melodies of the ragas amplify the frequency of the time of day, shifting your frequency into nature's vibration. Try the sunrise raga instead of a cup of coffee, the midday raga to help you digest lunch, the sunset raga to help you sleep, and any appropriate raga to help you recover from an illness. Be sure to listen for at least ten minutes, without interruption, while focusing only on the sound.

Imagine, instead of having two martinis at home after battling congested traffic, you listen to the sunset raga. Effortlessly your brain shifts from overstimulated erratic brain waves into an orderly, calmer rhythm. As the music washes through you, it brings your whole body into an alpha state, providing deep rest for all your organs. Listening to ragas is like being transported from an electrical storm into a warm breeze.

Ragas have been tested and shown to calm the nervous system and increase alpha brain waves associated with a relaxed, alert state of mind. You may be able to find healing ragas in Indian shops or large music stores with well-stocked foreign music sections. In addition Dr. Deepak Chopra's company also sells recordings of ragas composed for the three individual doshas. This and other mail-order sources for ragas are listed in the Appendix.

TOUCH: MASSAGE THERAPY

The sense of smell may be underappreciated, but in the United States the sense of touch is appallingly neglected. We are brought up to be leery of touching one another, and of touching ourselves. Touch not only can unleash a powerful and positive wave of emotion, it is an absolute requirement for good health. Without regular touching, newborn animals, including humans, fail to thrive. Massage, which is a form of touch, can relieve depression and anxiety, lower stress hormones in the blood, improve sleep, enhance the immune system, and make us more alert. Even simply holding the hand of a heart patient has been known to lower the heart rate. As Drs. Ornstein and Sobel write in Healthy Pleasures, "We speak of something being 'touching,' implying a close link between touch and the emotional reactions of the heart. It's more than a metaphor—our skin does speak to our hearts. And our hearts respond."

THE A-Z GUIDE

How Touch Affects the Doshas

The power of touch begins at the skin, through which life as we know it flows back and forth. The skin is the largest organ of the body; if stretched out flat, it would cover twenty square feet! In each inch of skin there are approximately nine feet of blood vessels and nine thousand nerve endings. The skin is the most intricate network of nerves in the human body, the main link between the outer world and our inner environment. Imagine, every hair on your body is connected to a nerve that makes its way along a great highway to your brain. (Try touching the tip of one of the hairs on your arm—your mind-body will be able to detect even this delicate a perturbation.)

Since skin is so nerve-rich, it is intimately connected with the vata dosha, the dosha that governs the nervous system and the one that all the other doshas follow. Because of its electrical nature, it is essential to lubricate the skin and mucous membranes with oils to insulate the electrical nerve impulses. Oils penetrate the skin and the entire nervous system, nourishing the beauty within and bringing radiant beauty to the skin surface.

Ayurveda has identified 108 specific points, called marmas, which are extremely sensitive and crucial for maintaining balanced doshas. Similar to acupuncture points, marma points are believed to be where the physical body meets the mind. Anatomically speaking, marma points are seen as nerve crossings—places where the nerves meet the fascia, or the sheet of connective tissue that covers or holds together body structures.

Many of them are also located over the lymph nodes. The lymph nodes are part of your lymphatic system. All your cells are bathed in lymphatic fluid, which brings nutrients to the cells and cleanses the tissues and organs of waste products and foreign materials, which are carried to the lymph nodes where they are destroyed. Exercise improves the lymph circulation, as does Ayurvedic massage, by increasing the flow of lymph through the lymph vessels. This form of massage improves immune function. It also raises serotonin levels in the brain, a neurotransmitter

AYURVEDA

that has a relaxing effect; it also increases other hormones secreted by the pineal gland. Known as door receptors, marma points are accessible through the skin.

How to Use Massage Therapy

In addition to the ability to lubricate, abhyanga (sesame oil massage, see Chapter 3) contacts marma points directly, and yoga gently stretches them. There are internal marmas, too, which are mentally stimulated during meditation. Another way to stimulate the marmas is through application of certain medicinal oils containing specific herbs. Massage and marma therapy with therapeutic oil is a mainstay of Ayurveda and is available at Ayurveda clinics. You can stimulate some points, as suggested in the A–Z listings, using the following oils, available by mail from the resources listed in the Appendix:

- Mahagenesh contains many herbs in a sesame oil base and is recommended for all doshas. After applying to the back of your neck and forehead, you'll feel energized.

- Neem is sesame oil with leaves of the neem tree added. It is used in India as a multipurpose oil effective for healing chronic and acute lesions and for use as a sunscreen and an insecticide. We have used it in our practice for many years and has seen a wide range of skin complaints cured completely by applying Neem. It is particularly good for soothing pitta problems.

- Brahmi is gotu kola herb in a coconut oil base. This may be used for daily abhyanga massage, but it also works wonders for people with sleep problems when applied to the forehead, soles of the feet, and around the belly button before retiring.

- Bhringhraj is a sweet-smelling sesame-based oil that rejuvenates, cools, and stabilizes pitta. Applying this oil during abhyanga nourishes and enlivens the sense of touch.

CHAPTER SIX
YOUR DAILY LIFESTYLE REGIMEN: PUTTING IT ALL TOGETHER

As in love, comedy, and skipping rope, timing is the key to success in Ayurveda. This chapter shows you how to structure your day so that you get the most benefit from the practices explained in chapters 3, 4, and 5. Although everyone, regardless of his or her dominant dosha, follows the same basic routine, as you'll see, each dosha has its own special timing for certain daily activities such as eating, exercising, and working. By following these few simple guidelines for integrating Ayurvedic practices into your life, you will begin to create a healthy mental and physical ecology in which every part of you takes care of itself without much further intervention. Making these general changes in your lifestyle will help balance your doshas and get to the root of any symptoms you may be experiencing. They reinforce the effects of the remedies suggested in the A—Z section and, with continued use, should prevent new or old symptoms from taking hold.

These practices act synergistically, so we encourage you to incorporate as many as you can to get the greatest benefit. However, you'll probably want to begin by incorporating just a few practices into your normal daily life and then gradually add more. We know how difficult it can be to break out of established habits and replace them with new ones. But even small changes can have a profound effect, providing you with the motivation to make further changes.

The goal is not, however, to become a slave to a rigid routine. Rather, the goal is to arrange your life so that it has a consistency and regularity and lays a stable foundation from which you can launch a rich and varied

AYURVEDA

life. To do this, you will probably need to reconsider your priorities and get up earlier to give yourself enough time to accomplish your morning practices. Until now you may have focused like a laser beam on getting to work on time; perhaps you also need to get your kids ready for school. It may seem impractical to squeeze in an unhurried breakfast, let alone meditation, yoga, and a daily massage. However, you'll find that if you make time for these practices, you'll sleep and use time more efficiently, be better prepared to face the day, have more energy, and be more productive. As Deepak Chopra writes in Perfect Health, "You gain more time than you lose, and it is quality time."

Once your doshas become more balanced and you feel calm, alert, energized, and happy, don't give in to the temptation to let your regimen slip. The benefits are cumulative and increase with long-term use, which is the only way to reach long-standing, deep-seated disorders. One longtime sufferer of chronic fatigue immune syndrome (CFIDS) discovered that "Everything that Dr. Thomas prescribed—herbs, diet, yoga, meditation, five-sense therapy—has made a noticeable difference in my health. If I stop doing any one of these things, I don't feel as well. Most people with CFIDS find that not much helps, or that some things help only for a while. Ayurveda continues to help me. And since I am able to do many things on my own at home, I have a renewed sense of power and control that has been lacking for the past twenty years."

TIMING, RHYTHM, AND THE DOSHAS

In Ayurveda what you do is important—but so is when you do it. Since ancient times Ayurveda has appreciated the health-building effects of being in sync with the rhythms of nature. The ancient belief that eating, sleeping, and working are best accomplished at certain limes of day and night is gaining support thanks to modern-day chronobiology, the study of the natural peaks and valleys in the metabolic cycle. Chronobiology is discovering that hormones, enzymes, and neurotransmitters all ebb and flow at predictable times during a twenty-four-hour day. As a result you

THE A-Z GUIDE

are better able to process information, perform certain tasks, digest food, and so on, during certain times. Even drugs can have markedly different effects depending on the time of day they are administered. Studies have shown that asthma attacks are most likely to occur in the middle of the night, the risk of stroke is greatest between six and ten A.M., and premenstrual syndrome appears to be related to changes in sleep patterns and exposure to light that affect a woman's biological clock.

The science of chronobiology is also proving that many tendencies are not just conditioning or habit. For hundreds of thousands of years humans have awakened and retired with the sun; as is the case with other living things, research shows that we are genetically programmed to function best when we go with the flow of daily and seasonal cycles.

Ayurveda explains this through the concept of daily dosha cycles: vata, pitta, and kapha are each at their peak during certain times of the day. Ayurveda divides the twenty-four-hour day into the following time periods (they are approximate because they depend on the season and geographic location):

Kapha times: 6 to 10 A.M.; 6 to 10 P.M.
Pitta times: 10 A.M. to 2 P.M.; 10 P.M. to 2 A.M.
Vata times: 2 to 6 A.M.; 2 to 6 P.M.

The Daily Lifestyle Regimens are based on this concept. For example morning is the kapha time of day, when the body feels slow, heavy, and calm. So everyone should be up by six A.M. or sunrise, because otherwise you find yourself too deeply in the kapha period and it will be difficult to get up and start the day. The middle of the day has pitta characteristics of activity and energy; this is when people naturally work most efficiently and are best able to digest food. So this is when you should eat your biggest meal of the day. The early afternoon is the vata period, which studies have shown is a time when most people exhibit the vata traits of thinking quickly and have the greatest manual dexterity. And starting at ten o'clock at night, the pitta metabolism is doing most of

AYURVEDA

its work, so you need to rest the body so that it can digest everything that happened that day. If you eat or engage in intense mental or physical activity late at night, you are swimming against the tide of your natural cycles. If you stay up late, you eventually get a "second wind" as pitta energy is diverted away from digesting food and the experiences of the day.

However, burning the midnight oil throws off your exquisitely calibrated biological clock. Your body organs become unduly fatigued and you feel tired, no matter how late you sleep the next morning. Even while you're sleeping, your physiology is busy. Between two and six A.M. body purification is preeminent, and it is vata that initiates the movement that promotes this. For example the small intestine contracts, emptying its contents into the large intestine; the liver is at peak efficiency in purifying and cleaning out the ama; and the kidney is processing the day's food and thoughts and moving them through the system.

Ayurveda also divides the year into seasons. In India there are six seasons. When these are translated into Western culture, the year is divided as follows:

> **Kapha Season:** Late winter through early spring
> (or when it is cold and wet)
> **Pitta Season:** Late spring through summer
> (or when it is hot)
> **Vata Season:** Fall and early winter
> (or when it is cold and wet)

What all this means is that people with a predominantly vata constitution (prakruti) will be especially sensitive during the vata times of day and the vata season. To avoid aggravating their vata, they should make a special effort to follow the vata-stabilizing diet and lifestyle during the vata season. The same holds true for pitta constitutions, and for kapha as well.

During transitions between the seasons, you aim to blend the regimens and the foods. It is also traditional to undergo rejuvenation practices between the seasons as you shift from the old energy to the new energy. A four or five-day Juice-and-Soup Fast is especially recommended during these times.

VATA: DAILY LIFESTYLE REGIMEN

	Basic	Additional
Early Morning	Arise by sunrise, without alarm clock Drink warm water Urinate and have bowel movement Brush teeth and scrape tongue Meditate Do sesame oil massage Do yoga Sun Salutation Do calming exercises such as tai chi or yoga, between six and ten A.M. or six and ten P.M.	Gargle with sesame oil Dry Massage twice a week Do additional yoga postures Do breathing exercises

AYURVEDA

	Bathe/shower with warm water	
	Eat breakfast by eight A.M. Take short walk	
	Midmorning Do active work; best time for meetings, communicating with others, doing chores and errands	
	Take short walk	
Midmorning	Do active work; best time for meetings, communicating with others, chores and errands	
Afternoon	Eat lunch between twelve and one	
	Low-key work: thinking, contemplation, reflect on the day	
	Vata tea break at four P.M.	
	Continue active work	
Evening	Evening Eat dinner between six and seven P. M.	Breathing exercises
	Take short walk	
	Engage in light, relaxing activity	Aromatherapy
	Meditate Go to bed by ten P.M.	Yoga

THE A-Z GUIDE

PITTA: DAILY LIFESTYLE REGIMEN

	Basic	Additional
Early Morning	Arise by sunrise, without alarm clock Drink warm water Urinate and have bowel movement Brush teeth and scrape tongue Meditate Do sesame oil massage Do yoga Sun Salutation Do exercise that is competitive and/or involves other people before ten A.M. or between six and ten P.M. Bathe/shower with warm	Gargle with sesame oil Dry Massage twice a week Do additional yoga postures Do breathing exercises

AYURVEDA

	water Eat breakfast by eight A.M. Take short walk	
Midmorning	Midmorning Do active work; best time for communicating with others, creative activities, nonstressful work in late morning	
Afternoon	Eat lunch between twelve and one Take short walk Do detailed work, communications, meetings, present creative ideas, make presentations and proposals Pitta tea break and snack at three P.M. Assess your performance and effectiveness, plan tomorrow's schedule	
Evening	Evening Eat dinner between six and seven P. M. Take short walk Engage in light, relaxing activity Meditate Go to bed by ten P.M.	Breathing exercises Aromatherapy Yoga

KAPHA: DAILY LIFESTYLE REGIMEN

	Basic	Additional
Early Morning	Arise by sunrise, without alarm clock; preferably earlier Drink warm water Urinate and have bowel movement Brush teeth and scrape tongue Meditate Do dry massage Do yoga Sun Salutation Do exercise that is competitive and/or involves other people before ten A.M. or between six and ten P.M. Bathe/shower with warm water	Do additional yoga postures Do breathing exercises

AYURVEDA

	Eat breakfast by eight A.M. Take short walk Take short walk	
Midmorning	Activities that require thinking, attend meetings	
Afternoon	Eat lunch between twelve and one Take short walk Resume work activities, especially those that involving light physical effort Kapha tea break and snack at three P.M. Continue active work	
Evening	Eat dinner between six and seven P. M. Do strenuous exercise such as walking uphill Engage in consistent stimulating activity outside the home, with wind down Meditate Go to bed by ten P.M.	Breathing exercises Aromatherapy Yoga

THE A-Z GUIDE

VATA-BALANCING GUIDELINES

Most Important

It's most important for this dosha in particular to maintain a regular daily schedule. This is difficult for vata people to accomplish, but it is absolutely necessary if they want to have more reliable energy and to sleep better. Once they start feeling better, it's tempting to push themselves and slip back into their old irregular habits—they should resist! They need to avoid becoming overstimulated; to include periods of rest, relaxation, and reflection (even if it's only fifteen minutes twice a day), particularly in the afternoon, when vata tends to become scattered; and to eat regular meals. They should be mindful of moving too much, doing too many things at one time, and thinking too much and too fast. Vata types usually get the least amount of sleep but need the most in order to rest their wound-up, overworked nervous systems. They should get a solid seven to eight hours of sleep and can sleep a little later than other doshas; they should go to bed early and rise at the same time every morning—even on the weekends.

Season

Fall is the season when vata is most prevalent, so they should be aware that this is when most imbalances occur—and be prepared. Vata types don't do well in rainy, damp, or windy weather, so they should stay out of the cold and avoid these conditions.

Food

Vata types should emphasize sweet, bitter, sour, heavy, oily, hot, vata-stabilizing foods and herbs, especially during fall and winter, the vata time of year. They should drink warm teas and fluids, and avoid caffeine and alcohol.

AYURVEDA

PITTA-BALANCING GUIDELINES

Most Important

Pitta types are usually highly organized; they often need to loosen up and do things just for fun rather than because of a desire to reach a particular goal. They need to tone down their activities after six P.M.; evening meditation is especially useful for calming the pitta mind. Balanced pitta types can manage with six hours of sleep because they have the most natural energy of all the doshas. But they need to avoid overexertion, which can burn out their fire, and be sure to allow time to relax and rejuvenate and to spend time in nature.

Season

Pitta is predominant in the late spring through summer, and pitta types are therefore imbalanced by hot, humid weather and conditions. They need to avoid overexposure to heat and direct sun.

Food

Pitta types should emphasize sweet, bitter, astringent, cold, heavy, oily, pitta-cooling foods and herbs, especially during the late spring and summer. They should eat whenever they are hungry, and not skip meals. They should avoid stimulating foods and herbs, especially artificial stimulants and drugs.

KAPHA-BALANCING GUIDELINES

Most Important

Kapha types should maintain a strict, structured schedule to avoid lethargy and inertia. However, to avoid getting stuck in a rut, they need to introduce some slight change into their routine every day. They

THE A-Z GUIDE

should engage in vigorous exercise every day and eat a very light breakfast, if any, and a light supper. Kapha types usually get the most sleep, but require the least. They should rise the earliest of all three types because they tend to sluggishness; getting more than six to seven hours a night makes it harder for them to get going in the morning. The early-to-bed and early-to-rise rule is especially relevant for kapha types, and they must avoid staying in bed after six A.M. at all costs.

Season

Late winter and early spring is when kapha is feeling most lethargic, and they need to strongly resist this influence by committing to an active life at this time. Kaphas are adversely affected by the cold, damp weather prevalent at this time, so it's best that they make an effort to keep warm and avoid these conditions.

Food

Kapha types should emphasize bitter, astringent, pungent, light, dry, hot, kapha-stabilizing foods and herbs, reduce sugars and sweets, and drink warming teas and fluids.

AYURVEDA

PART TWO

THE A-Z GUIDE TO COMMON CONDITIONS AND HOW TO TREAT THEM WITH AYURVEDA

In this section you will learn how to treat more than sixty common conditions naturally, by applying specific Ayurvedic practices and remedies to balance your doshas. We have divided the prescriptive advice into three categories: We begin with general recommendations, then provide herbal remedies, and finally, therapies that will delight all five of your senses. While any one category of approach will have some effect, you will obtain the greatest relief if you use all three together.

Follow the prescriptive advice until the symptoms subside. Ideally you should practice the appropriate dosha balancing daily routine outlined in Chapter 6 as the first step in creating a foundation for healing and prevention of future episodes of this symptom. However, we realize that some people will just want to treat the symptom that is bothering them.

AYURVEDA

Ayurveda can be effectively used this way, but if symptoms persist, it's probably due to an underlying imbalance that needs to be addressed via daily routines that include rising and going to bed early, meditation, physical activity, and dietary practices.

For a more detailed explanation of the general recommendations, refer to Chapter 3, which discusses . . .

- General lifestyle recommendations
- Diet and eating habits
- Exercise
- Oil massage (abhyanga)
- Dry massage (garshana)
- Nasal-passage lubrication (nasaya)
- Breathing practices (pranayama)
- Meditation
- Yoga

For a more detailed explanation of food as medicine and herbal remedies, refer to Chapter 4, which discusses . . .

- Food guidelines for balancing vata, pitta, and kapha
- Herbs and spices for cooking and making teas
- How to use herbs and spices medicinally
- Recipes for ghee, Ten-Day Ginger Treatment, Juice and-Soup Fast, copper water, and kicharee

For detailed instructions on various five-sense therapies and on how to make churna, refer to Chapter 5.

And for Daily Lifestyle Regimens appropriate for balancing vata, pitta, and kapha, refer to Chapter 6.

THE A-Z GUIDE

ABDOMINAL BLOATING

Abdominal bloating, when the abdomen distends and there may be intestinal or abdominal gas, is the cardinal sign of dysfunction of the agni, the digestive fire, and is usually caused by a vata imbalance. In Ayurveda we describe it as the first sign of an imbalance in the "gastrointestinal consciousness." Bloating occurs when the gastrointestinal tract is unable to split food into the smallest particles and release the nourishing enzymes into the system. Also see Indigestion.

AYURVEDIC SELF-CARE

Follow the appropriate Daily Lifestyle Regimen for your dosha, paying particular attention to your diet and eating habits.

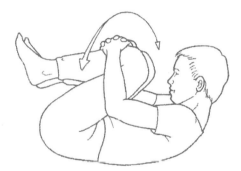

Rocking and Rolling: Sit on the floor and pull both legs up to your chest; interlock your hands over your knees. Roll your body backward and forward, ten times in each direction, keeping your elbows close to your legs.

Eat a light diet of primarily vegetables and rice, or kicharee; the Ten-Day Ginger Treatment is also recommended. There are several yoga movements that release wind and gases from the body, including toe bending, ankle bending, ankle rotation, hand clenching, wrist bending, leg rotations, and the posture known as Rocking and Rolling.

AYURVEDA

HERBAL REMEDIES

- Triphala treats the entire digestive tract. Take 1/2 teaspoon triphala mixed with 1/2 cup warm water every evening at bedtime.

FIVE-SENSE THERAPIES

- Taste: Emphasize sweet, sour, bitter, and salty foods, spices, and herbs. Consuming the summer churna with a little salt and lemon flakes is an easy way to get all these tastes in the appropriate proportions.

- Smell: Use warm, sweet, and sour essential-oil aromas, such as rose, cloves, cinnamon, basil, and orange.

- Sight: Green and blue are recommended to relieve bloating.

- Hearing: Listen to the midmorning raga between ten A.M. and one P.M. or the midday raga between one and four P.M.

- Touch: Apply a drop of warm sesame oil and pressure to the marma point known as Oorvee.

THE A-Z GUIDE

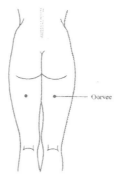

The manna point for abdominal bloating: Oorvee.

IMPORTANT PRECAUTIONS FOR ABDOMINAL BLOATING

See a health professional if abdominal bloating persists is accompanied by severe discomfort and pain, which may indicate a possible obstruction of the bowel, a serious condition.

ABDOMINAL PAIN

Pain can occur in many locations of the large area known as the abdomen. Much abdominal pain is due to indigestion, which has symptoms such as heartburn, nausea, burping, and intestinal gas, sometimes accompanied by pain. For additional information, see Indigestion. Here we are concerned with what is medically known as left epigastric pain, in which the discomfort is located on the left side, under the rib cage. Pain in this area is specifically associated with the stomach. Sharp abdominal pain is the number-one sign for a vata imbalance; burning pain is due to aggravated pitta, and dull pain characterizes kapha imbalance.

AYURVEDA

AYURVEDIC SELF-CARE

Follow the appropriate Daily Lifestyle Regimen for your dosha, paying particular attention to your diet and eating habits. Eat a light diet of primarily vegetables and rice, or kicharee and the Ten-Day Ginger Treatment. The Leg Cycling Pose is particularly useful for relieving this condition.

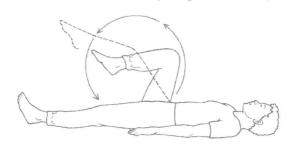

Leg Cycling Pose: Lie flat on your back and raise your right leg. First, make ten forward-cycling movements and ten reverse-cycling movements. Repeat with your left leg. Second, if you have enough abdominal strength to prevent your lower back from popping up, use both legs to make alternating cycling movements, ten times in both directions. Third, keep your legs pressed together and again make ten cycling motions in each direction. It will help to tuck your palms under your buttocks. Repeat the first and third movements, making big sideways circles instead of cycling.

HERBAL REMEDIES

Use one of the following when you experience abdominal pain:

- Combine 5 parts shatavari (Asparagus racemosus), 3 parts guduchi (Tinospora cordifolia), and 2 parts kama dudha; take 1/4 teaspoon of this mixture daily in 1/2 cup warm water following lunch and dinner.

- Take 1/2 teaspoon amalaki (Emblica officinalis) before bedtime every night, mixed with 1/2 cup warm water.

THE A-Z GUIDE

- Make a paste using 1/2 teaspoon fresh grated ginger and 1 teaspoon ghee; apply over the area of discomfort; leave on for 20 minutes, or apply before going to bed and leave on overnight.

FIVE-SENSE THERAPIES

- Taste: Bitter is better for digestion, so emphasize foods, herbs, and spices that have a bitter taste; some people also benefit from sweet and sour tastes as well. •

- Smell: Use aromatherapy with sweet, bitter, and cool aromas, such as sandalwood, cinnamon, and jasmine.

- Sight: Choose yellow-green or blue-green colors.

- Hearing: Play the midmorning raga between the hours of ten A.M. and one P.M.

- Touch: Apply one drop of warm sesame oil and finger pressure to the marma point known as Oorvee.

IMPORTANT PRECAUTIONS FOR ABDOMINAL PAIN

Seek medical care if: the pain is severe; the pain begins near the navel and then moves to the lower right abdomen (a possible sign of appendicitis); the pain is severely disabling; you have vomiting or diarrhea that is persistent or contains blood; or there is a possibility of poisoning.

AYURVEDA

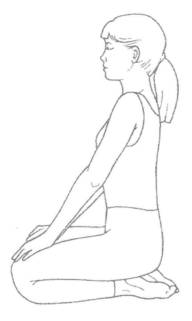

Thunderbolt Pose: This is especially effective after a meal. Kneel with your knees apart and feet stretched back; your heels are not touching but your big toes are crossed. Lower yourself down so that your buttocks rest on the soles of your feet. Hold for at least five minutes, with eyes closed, and breathing normally.

ACID STOMACH

Acid stomach is often a result of indigestion. If you have poor digestion, you compromise the absorption and assimilation of food. According to Ayurveda, your digestive system begins to increase the digestive liquid and fire to compensate, and your system becomes overheated. As a result you have high pitta and this creates acidity in the stomach.

Also see Indigestion.

THE A-Z GUIDE

AYURVEDIC SELF-CARE

Follow the appropriate Daily Lifestyle Regimen for your dosha, paying particular attention to your diet and eating habits. The yoga pose Thunderbolt is particularly useful for relieving acid stomach.

HERBAL REMEDIES

- Take 1/2 teaspoon shatavari (Asparagus racemosus) mixed with 1/2 cup warm water or milk before eating; and 1 cup fennel tea three times a day until the acidity is relieved.

FIVE-SENSE THERAPIES

- Taste: Bitter and astringent foods, herbs, and spices reduce acidity; it may be helpful to use the summer churna plus a little salt and lemon flakes every day.

- Smell: Use aromatherapy with sweet, cool aromas, such as sandalwood, jasmine, cinnamon, and fennel.

- Sight: Use yellow if your problem is related to feelings of anger or rage. Use blue if the acidity is related to lack of communication of suppressed emotions such as grief or sadness.

- Hearing: Listen to the midmorning raga between the hours of ten A.M. and one P.M.

- Touch: Apply one drop of coconut oil and slight finger pressure to the marma point known as Oorvee.

AYURVEDA

IMPORTANT PRECAUTIONS FOR ACID STOMACH

Don't put up with an acid stomach; if symptoms don't subside within one week of Ayurvedic treatment, consult a physician. This symptom could indicate an ulcer or preulcerous condition.

ACNE

Most people consider acne to be the bane of adolescence, but it can also happen to adults, even those who went through their teens blemish-free. In teenagers acne may plague otherwise healthy kids and so is considered an acute condition. However, in Ayurveda adult acne is considered to be a superficial sign of important underlying imbalance of the pitta dosha.

The signs of acne—red, inflamed pimples; whiteheads; blackheads— occur when oil glands produce too much oil (sebum) or oil that contains ama, the toxic byproducts of poorly digested food such as junk food. Bacteria on the skin interact with the sebum and cause abscesses to form—inflammation and plugging up of the hair follicles near the glands. Infection may set in which can eventually cause scars.

If you have mild acne with only a few intermittent eruptions, follow the general suggestions for Ayurvedic self-care and try one of the Ayurvedic remedies. Severe cases require professional Ayurvedic evaluation and care.

AYURVEDIC SELF-CARE

Acne is usually a sign of a pitta imbalance, so follow the Daily Lifestyle Regimen for pitta, paying particular attention to stress-reducing practices such as meditation, abdominal breathing and yoga. The Sun Salutations and the Lion yoga pose are particularly helpful. Also be sure to keep your

THE A-Z GUIDE

skin clean, but overenthusiastic scrubbing may actually worsen acne. Avoid squeezing pimples, since this can spread infection and injure delicate, inflamed tissues.

HERBAL REMEDIES

- Turmeric is antibiotic and antibacterial. Form a paste of 1/4 teaspoon turmeric powder with a little water; carefully apply to blemishes with a cotton swab—turmeric will stain clothes.

- You may also wash your face in the morning using chickpea powder mixed with water to make a paste; apply to your skin like a lotion and rub gently before rinsing off.

- Apply a light coating of Neem oil before retiring.

- Take 1/2 teaspoon manjistha (Rubio cordifolium) with pitta tea three times a week to purify the blood.

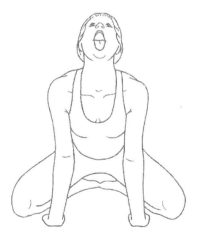

Lion Pose: Sit on your feet, knees apart, facing the sun if possible. Place your hands on the floor between your knees, with the fingertips pointing toward your body. Lean forward, keeping your arms

straight and tilting your head back. Open your eyes wide as you open your mouth and stick out your tongue as far as possible, exhaling with an ah sound the length of your exhalation.

FIVE-SENSE THERAPIES

- Taste: Emphasize foods, herbs, and spices that are bitter, sweet, and astringent; using the summer churns every day is a simple, easy way to use taste therapy.

- Smell: Use aromatherapy that is warm, sweet, sour, and bitter, such as a combination of orange, sandalwood, and mint.

- Sight: Color therapy consists of yellow-orange and green; also look in the mirror and deliberately smile at your image for 60 seconds every morning.

- Hearing: Listen to soft, gentle, classical music generally, and avoid hard, electric, pounding music. Ragas composed for the sunrise time of day (seven to ten A.M.) and late afternoon (four to seven P.M.) are also helpful.

- Touch: Tap your temples gently to calm your thought process; pull your earlobes to stimulate the immune system.

IMPORTANT PRECAUTIONS FOR ACNE

Seek medical care if the condition is severe or if the following signs appear in an adult: general illness such as weight change, change in hair distribution, change in the menstrual cycle, change in general energy or body temperature.

THE A-Z GUIDE

ALLERGIES

According to some allergists, half of all disease is due to allergies. An allergy is commonly defined as a reaction of the immune system to something in your environment. A healthy immune system recognizes and destroys potentially harmful foreign infectious invaders such as bacteria and viruses, or noninfectious irritants such as pollen, dust, or animal dander. An allergic person reacts more strongly than usual to these substances and to others such as certain foods, molds, medicines, or chemicals. Many body systems may suffer from symptoms, but the nose, sinuses, throat, and other parts of the respiratory tract as well as the skin and digestive system are especially vulnerable.

The Ayurvedic system doesn't emphasize a precise diagnosis; rather it sees the allergic condition as a breakdown in the digestive process. The accumulation of ama, or waste, clogs the channels of the body and your nervous, hormonal, and immune systems miscommunicate. This leads to a generalized state of alarm in the body. Sticky ama, a sluggish digestive fire, and an overtaxed immune system open the door to a bacterial invasion and overstimulation of the antigen-antibody response. Eventually the immune system becomes exhausted. According to Ayurveda, pitta and vata are more susceptible to allergies than kapha types.

Complete cure for recurrent or chronic allergies requires professional treatment by a health professional trained in Ayurveda. We usually begin treatment with desensitization to the offending substances. This is accompanied by clearing up of ama through proper diet and food combining, increasing the digestive fire, and restoring the immune system with herbs and five-sense therapy. However, you may be able to treat acute attacks and reduce symptoms with self-care. What follows are common Ayurvedic remedies for allergies in general. For remedies for specific types of allergies, also see Skin Rash/Hives, Dermatitis/Eczema, Hay Fever, and Electronic Pollution. Asthma, which has a variety of possible causes including allergic reaction, has its own section.

AYURVEDA

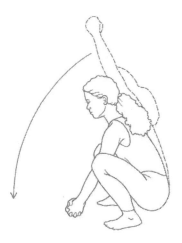

Chopping Wood: Squat down, with your feet flat on the floor and your knees apart. Inhale and clasp your hands together overhead; keeping your arms straight, exhale as you make a chopping motion as if you were cutting wood with an ax. Repeat ten or twenty times. Do this slowly, with conscious awareness of each part of your body and its movement.

AYURVEDIC SELF-CARE

Since allergies are due to low agni, or digestive fire, follow the appropriate Daily Lifestyle Regimen for your dosha, paying particular attention to practices that increase agni, the digestive fire, such as the Ten-Day Ginger Treatment. Eat food that is hot in temperature rather than cold. Sun Salutation is an excellent therapy for allergy, and the Chopping Wood yoga movement is particularly useful for relieving this condition.

HERBAL REMEDIES

- Drink 1 cup copper water daily upon arising; then add one of the following remedies until symptoms subside:

THE A-Z GUIDE

- Combine 1 pinch black pepper with 1 tablespoon ghee; take internally or apply directly to skin rash once a day.

- Add 1/4 teaspoon each of powdered cumin and coriander to 1 cup milk and heat until lukewarm; drink once a day.

- Combine equal parts each of shatavari (Asparagus racemosus) and guduchi (Tinospora cordifolia); add 1/4 teaspoon of the mixture to warm water and drink three times a day.

- Add 1/2 teaspoon triphala to 1/2 cup warm water and drink at bedtime; continue this treatment for three months.

FIVE-SENSE THERAPIES

- Taste: Emphasize foods, spices, and herbs that are sweet, bitter, and astringent; the summer churna will provide these tastes.

- Smell: Use aromatherapy with oils that are sweet, bitter, and astringent, particularly bergamot, mint, and lavender.

- Sight: Favor the color orange.

- Hearing: Listen to baroque music, or to the midmorning raga between the hours of ten A.M. and one P.M.

AYURVEDA

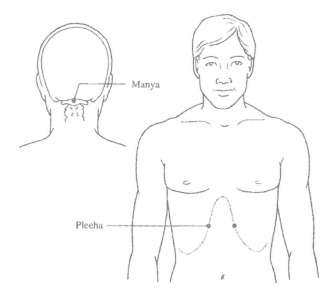

The marma points for allergies: Manya and Pleeha.

• Touch: Apply one drop of warm sesame oil and finger pressure to the marma points known as Pleeha and Manya, shown above.

IMPORTANT PRECAUTIONS FOR ALLERGIES

Consult a health care professional if allergies persist despite Ayurvedic self-care, or if there is wheezing or trouble breathing.

THE A-Z GUIDE

ANGER

Ayurveda teaches that basic survival needs are the foundation of all emotions. Anger is a very useful instinctual emotion that arises from the frustration of a basic need not being met. Up to a certain point it is positive and healthy to feel and express your anger, because it indicates you have the will to live. However, it does have its consequences, whether you are the one who is angry or the one to whom the anger is directed. It is important to express anger in a constructive rather than a destructive way.

Vata, pitta, and kapha types all experience anger. However, this emotion is usually attributed to a pitta imbalance since the elements of fire and water are at play when anger is expressed. Fiery enzymes and digestive juices are either overstimulated or understimulated in a person who tends to become angry frequently. Therefore it stands to reason that physiologically you need to regulate the digestive system. Emotionally you need to explore the basic needs that you feel are not being met. Attachment, a kapha trait, is another aspect of anger: If you are so set on having it one way and it just isn't going that way, letting go and acceptance is the antidote.

Ayurveda can help you deal with anger, whether it expresses itself as a screaming match with your boss, your spouse, your parent, your teenager, or your friend. Such angry encounters can leave us shaking with indignation, sleepless, and obsessive about the conversation for days afterward ("I should have said . . ."). You may feel angry with yourself for having yelled back, or perhaps remorse over things you said or did. These are normal reactions and part of the healing process. Such acute reactions will subside naturally; they are not to be confused with those of the chronically angry person who is abusive and volatile in social situations.

AYURVEDA

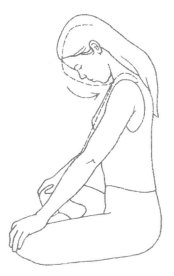

Chin Lock: Sit in a cross-legged position that allows your knees to touch the floor, or stand with legs hip-width apart and knees slightly bent. Place your palms on your knees, close your eyes, and relax your body. Inhale and bend your head forward so that your chin is pressed tightly against your chest. Straighten your arms and hunch your shoulders up. Hold this pose for as long as you can comfortably hold your breath. Exhale, relax your shoulders, and lift your head. Rest, and repeat up to ten times.

AYURVEDIC SELF-CARE

Follow the appropriate Daily Lifestyle Regimen for your dosha, paying particular attention to your tendency to anger during your meditation, and to deep breathing (pranayama). Writing about your feelings in a journal is particularly helpful during a crisis. Recognize that it is healthy to vent your anger, but it is also healthy to say you're sorry. The yoga movement shown are particularly useful for relieving stress, anxiety, and anger when performed after your other yoga postures and before meditation.

THE A-Z GUIDE

HERBAL REMEDIES

- Take 1/4 teaspoon shatavari (Asparagus racemosus) and 1/8 teaspoon saraswati (women) or 1/4 teaspoon ashwaghanda (Withania somnifera) and 1/8 teaspoon saraswati (men) in pitta tea morning and evening. Take for 2 weeks, then rest the system.

- Put 2 bunches of cilantro, 4 apples, and 1/2 teaspoon ginger through a juicer (this should yield 8 to 10 ounces). Take once a day, at lunchtime if possible.

FIVE-SENSE THERAPIES

- Taste: Emphasize foods, herbs, and spices that are sweet, bitter, and astringent, such as those found in summer churna.

- Smell: Use aromatherapy with sweet, cool aromas, such as sandalwood, mint, and jasmine.

- Sight: Indigo and blue help to cool feelings of anger.

- Hearing: Listen to soft, soothing classical music or the midmorning raga between the hours of ten A.M. and one P.M.

- Touch: Apply Brahmi oil to your forehead, the area around the navel, and the soles of your feet before retiring.

IMPORTANT PRECAUTIONS FOR ANGER

Sometimes professional help is needed to uproot the deep-seated causes of negative emotions. If you find you are frequently or automatically responding to situations with anger, consult a psychotherapist.

AYURVEDA

ANXIETY AND FEAR

Life is full of experiences that may cause some people to become temporarily fearful. Even people we consider to be psychologically strong and healthy may be prone to pre-exam jitters or pre-interview nerves; a person may fret about an upcoming wedding, giving a speech or presentation, or performing in a concert, play, or competition. In other cases a recent unanticipated frightening experience may shake you up for a while—a near-miss car accident or a natural disaster such as an earthquake, hurricane, flood, or fire.

You may become paralyzed with fear or not be able to stop shaking; you may think constantly about the future or past event, lose sleep, and be unable to concentrate, which makes dealing with the experience more difficult.

Ayurveda sees anxiety and fear as a classic vata imbalance. The electrical energy of vata becomes dehydrated, starts behaving like static electricity, and the mind acquires an unnecessary charge that is perceived as fear and anxiety. Ayurveda can soothe both adults and children through the emotional ill effects of such specific crises. Long-standing or chronic fear and free-floating anxiety, however, are deep-seated conditions and require professional evaluation.

AYURVEDIC SELF-CARE

Relaxation techniques are tools that help us consciously relax for a short period every day and can help calm fears. As you follow the appropriate Daily Lifestyle Regimen for your dosha, pay particular attention to meditation, exercise, yoga, and deep breathing. These are proven and effective ways to reach a state of relaxation—they are like taking a minivacation. Or you might want to try progressive muscle relaxation.

As with all symptoms, suppressing your fear is not healthy in the long run. Generally it is better to acknowledge your fear and talk to another person or persons in a safe, supportive environment. The right amount

THE A-Z GUIDE

of fear can actually help some people perform better, or stimulate their thinking about how to minimize fearful experiences in the future. The more important and deeper the feeling of fear, the more likely that unhealed fears in the past are being stirred up. But even this can be helpful because it brings up issues that are still bothering you and should be dealt with.

Listen to your own individual needs: Do you feel better when you are left alone, or when you are in the company of others? Do you find comfort in talking to people who share similar experiences and feelings? Can you find ways to distract yourself until the fear passes?

Progressive Muscle Relaxation

This is a simple, no-frills technique used to relax the mind-body by alternately tensing and relaxing the muscles. It may take about a half hour at first, but with time it becomes easier and you will achieve the relaxed state sooner. Make sure you are in quiet surroundings—no TV or radio playing, telephone unplugged or off the hook. Have the room temperature on the warm side; keep a blanket handy in case you feel chilly during the process. To begin, lie down on a comfortable surface, close your eyes, and take a few deep, slow breaths. Direct your attention to your right leg. Stretch it away from your body, pointing your foot hard; hold until it begins to tremble slightly and then let go and allow it to relax completely. Repeat with the left leg. Next move your attention to your right arm, stretch it and then let it go limp as you did with your leg. Clench your hand into a tight fist; hold and then release. Stretch the fingers out straight; hold and then release. Proceed to alternately contract and then relax the muscles of your hips (contract buttocks, then release), waist (pull in your stomach, then release), back (press your lower back to the floor, then release), chest (contract your ribs inward so that your chest becomes concave, then release), shoulders (scrunch them up toward your ears, then relax them back down), and scalp (wiggle your ears, move your eyebrows up and down, then release). Finally, move to your face: Open your mouth and eyes wide, next scrunch them in, then let the muscles go. Take a few deep, slow breaths (breathe

AYURVEDA

slowly and rhythmically throughout) and repeat the exercise. Then just lie still for ten minutes or so, allowing your mind to let go of whatever is bothering you. If thoughts enter, just let them float by without trying to stop them. When you are ready, stretch your arms overhead, point your feet, take a deep breath, and gradually open your eyes and return to your surroundings.

HERBAL REMEDIES

- Combine 1/4 teaspoon each of jatamansi (Nordostachys jatamansi) and Brahmi (gotu kola); take with 1 cup warm water twice a day.

FIVE-SENSE THERAPIES

- Taste: Emphasize sweet, sour, and salty tastes when choosing food, herbs, and spices. Sprinkling winter churna on your food every day will provide these tastes.

- Smell: Sweet, warm aromas, such as lavender, basil, orange, and clove calm vata and ease fear and anxiety.

- Sight: Green, yellow, or violet color therapy is also soothing.

- Hearing: Listening to Gregorian chants or the sunset raga between the hours of seven and ten P.M. stabilizes vata.

- Touch: Abhyanga massage with Brahmi oil is a general relaxant. You may also apply one drop of warm sesame oil and finger pressure to the marma point known as Manya.

IMPORTANT PRECAUTIONS FOR ANXIETY AND FEAR

Seek medical care if the symptoms of anxiety are accompanied by worsening or severe physical symptoms such as chest pain, abdominal pain, headache, difficulty breathing, or any other dramatic change in ability to function.

ARGUMENTATIVENESS

Argumentativeness is a sign of a pitta imbalance. While pitta's strength is its ability to discriminate, too much pitta will cause the mind to get stuck in a judgmental mode and tip toward too much discrimination. The mind becomes overheated, causing aggravation and the need to release the hot energy by becoming picky, disagreeable, and quarrelsome.

AYURVEDIC SELF-CARE

Following the appropriate Daily Lifestyle Regimen for your dosha on a long-term basis is the best approach for evening out intensities in your personality. In particular the yoga routine Sun Salutation oxygenates the system and helps release superficial stresses that can lead to argumentativeness; and meditation helps release the deeper stresses.

HERBAL REMEDIES

- Combine 1/4 teaspoon each saraswati and arjuna (Terminalia arjuna) with 1/2 teaspoon triphala; take V8 teaspoon of this mixture with warm water or a mild herb tea such as chamomile in the morning and evening. If you are very cranky, take 1/2 teaspoon.

- Taste: Choose sweet, bitter, and astringent foods, spices, and herbs; you'll find these tastes in the summer churna.

- Smell: Use sweet, cool aromas, such as sandalwood, rose, and mint.

- Sight: The colors indigo and blue-green help settle down the argumentative mind.

AYURVEDA

- Hearing: Listen to the midmorning raga between the hours of ten A.M. and one P.M.

- Touch: Massage your forehead, ears, and the bottom of your feet using Brahmi oil.

IMPORTANT PRECAUTIONS FOR ARGUMENTATIVENESS

Sometimes professional help is needed to uproot the deep-seated causes of negative behaviors. If you find you are frequently argumentative, consult a psychotherapist.

ARTHRITIS

Arthritis is actually an umbrella term for a number of joint diseases, in which one or more of the joints in your body become inflamed and painful. Arthritis can affect people of all ages, though it is most commonly troubling to older people. It varies in severity from mild aches and pains to severe impairment and joint deformity.

From an Ayurvedic point of view arthritis is both a physical and an emotional condition. Repressed, undigested emotions or metabolic ama accumulate throughout the body, but particularly the joints, causing symptoms. Degenerative arthritis is due primarily to a vata imbalance, and it is known as "wandering pain." It is often worsened by windy, cold weather. Inflammatory arthritis is due to a pitta imbalance, and rheumatoid arthritis arises from a kapha imbalance.

AYURVEDIC SELF-CARE

Follow the appropriate Daily Lifestyle Regimen for your dosha, making an extra effort to avoid foods in the nightshade family (tomatoes, white potatoes, peppers, and eggplant). Yoga is an excellent way to keep the

THE A-Z GUIDE

joints limber and lubricated. Before doing yoga, soak for 20 minutes in a warm bath to which you have added Epsom salts. You will also find deep breathing exercises (pranayama) to be profoundly relaxing.

HERBAL REMEDIES

For generalized arthritis, choose one of the following:

- A good general remedy for all doshas is to drink a tea made by combining 1 cup hot water with 1 teaspoon ground ginger and 2 tablespoons castor oil, which contains natural steroids. Drink in the early morning (kapha), midday (pitta), or evening (vata).

- Combine 1/2 teaspoon triphala and 1/2 teaspoon yogaraj guggulu with 1/2 cup warm water; take twice a day following lunch and dinner.

- Combine 5 parts ashwagandha (Withania somnifera), 2 parts trikatu, 3 parts bala (Sida cordifolia), and 2 parts garlic; mix 1/4 teaspoon of this mixture with kapha tea and drink twice a day following lunch and dinner.

For degenerative joints, choose one of the following:

- Take 1 teaspoon ashwagandha with 1 cup warm water, three times a day.

- Mix 1/4 teaspoon ashwagandha with 1 teaspoon ghee; rub on affected joints twice daily.

AYURVEDA

For rheumatoid arthritis, choose one of the following:

- Combine 1/8 teaspoon yogaraj guggulu with 1/4 teaspoon trikatu; take twice daily with kapha tea after meals.

- Take 1 tablespoon castor oil once a week to cleanse the system.

- Take 1 teaspoon each chitrak (Plumbago zeylonica), guduchi (Tinospora cordifolia), and turmeric with 1 cup warm water or vata tea three times a day.

For rheumatoid joints, choose one of the following:

- Combine 1/2 teaspoon each of ginger, black pepper, pippali (long pepper), and honey; take three times a day.

- Take 1/2 teaspoon triphala with 1/2 cup warm water.

FIVE-SENSE THERAPIES

- Taste: Sweet, bitter, and astringent foods, spices, and herbs are good for arthritis, so use the summer churna every day.

- Smell: Warm aromas such as clove, mint, and eucalyptus are helpful, especially if you add them to your bath water.

- Sight: Favor the colors red, orange, blue, and violet.

- Hearing: Listen to the sunset raga between the hours of seven and ten P.M. or the midday raga between one and four P.M.

- Touch: For general relief, apply mustard oil to the joints and massage with a circular motion before retiring. (To make your own mustard oil, combine 4 parts sesame oil with 1 part black mustard seed.) For vata related arthritis, apply castor oil to your joints and massage gently. For kapha-related arthritis, .do a silk-glove massage.

IMPORTANT PRECAUTIONS FOR ARTHRITIS

If pain persists or is accompanied by redness and inflammation, consult your physician.

ASTHMA

Asthma is a chronic condition that causes episodes of wheezing and shortness of breath. The symptoms are due to a temporary contraction in the muscles of the breathing passages, which swell and fill with mucus. The throat and chest feel tight, and you may cough and produce thick phlegm. Symptoms of asthma range from mild to severe and may come on suddenly and dramatically or gradually worsen with increasing difficulty breathing. An attack may be as brief as five minutes or last for days on end.

Since asthma is quite frightening and may cause death, sometimes it is so severe that allopathic drugs are appropriate and necessary in spite of Ayurvedic treatment. Commonly used drugs include ephedrine and steroids to relax the muscles of the constricted passageways, inhalers, and expectorants to clear the phlegm. These all have side effects and when used frequently or improperly they can lose their effectiveness and cause a person to be dependent on them.

An Ayurvedic practitioner can provide medicines that reduce the frequency and severity of this chronic, deep, and often genetically determined condition. Ayurvedic home care and remedies may ease the symptoms of an attack, but be sure to have the disease diagnosed professionally and understand your particular symptom pattern before attempting to treat asthma yourself.

AYURVEDA

Ayurveda recognizes three types of asthma:

- Vata-type asthma is worse in the evening and is characterized by dryness and coldness, spasms in the brachial tree, but no inflammation; it may be accompanied by constipation and intestinal gas.

- Pitta-type asthma appears at midday and is characterized by bronchitis, a burning pain in the chest, fever, nausea, vomiting, and irritability.

- Kapha-type asthma occurs in the early morning and late evening and is characterized by increased and plentiful bronchial secretions, profuse expectoration with wheezing, and is accompanied by a cough, runny nose, sinus congestion, sweaty hands and feet, and tears in the eyes.

AYURVEDIC SELF-CARE

Follow the appropriate Daily Lifestyle Regimen for your dosha, making sure you do the deep abdominal breathing exercises (pranayama) and yoga Sun Salutation, which are very helpful between attacks. The yoga position shown are particularly helpful for asthma. In addition regular vigorous exercise between attacks helps strengthen the lungs. Meditation is relaxing and can be helpful for prevention and can also be used at the onset of an attack to lessen symptoms. Drinking plenty of fluids helps loosen mucus and replace the water your body loses during the shallow rapid breathing and increased perspiration during an asthma attack. The following Ayurvedic remedies will also relieve the spasms of asthma; repeat every 2 hours if symptoms are acute and 4 hours if mild, until symptoms subside.

THE A-Z GUIDE

HERBAL REMEDIES

Take 1/2 teaspoon triphala mixed with 1/2 cup warm water daily at bedtime.

- Combine 4 parts sesame oil with 1 part black mustard seed to make mustard oil; apply to chest area.

- Mix with 1 cup hot water and drink as a tea: 1/2 teaspoon cinnamon, 1/3 teaspoon cardamom, 1/2 teaspoon fresh grated ginger, 1 teaspoon jaggery (brown sugar), and 1 pinch powdered clove.

- Combine 5 parts dashmoola, 3 parts ashwagandha (Withania somnifera), and 3 parts pippali (long pepper); take 1/4 teaspoon of this mixture with 1/2 cup boiled water twice daily following lunch and dinner.

FIVE-SENSE THERAPIES

- Taste: Emphasize foods, spices, and herbs that are sweet, sour, and salty; using the winter churna is a simple way to do this.

- Smell: Use aromatherapy with essentials oils that have a warm smell, such as cloves, eucalyptus, and lavender.

- Sight: Surround yourself with the colors green, yellow, and indigo.

- Hearing: Listen to the late-afternoon raga between the hours of four and seven P.M.

- Touch: Daily sesame oil massage (abhyanga) balances vata and thus helps lessen asthma. In addition you may

AYURVEDA

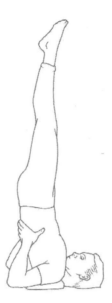

Shoulder Stand: Lie on your back, arms and hands flat against the floor, with one or two folded towels placed under your shoulders. Exhale, bend your knees, and slowly raise your legs and torso up. Simultaneously bend your elbows and place your hands near your waist to support your body. Straighten and extend your legs toward the ceiling. Breathe rhythmically and hold the pose as long as is comfortable, gradually increasing the length up to two minutes. (Note: Do not perform this posture if you have a chronic back problem or high blood pressure, or if your neck feels pinched.)

THE A-Z GUIDE

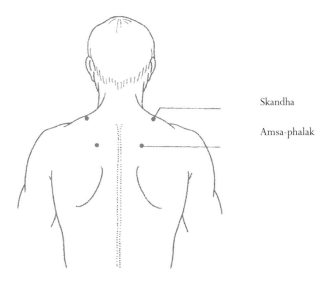

Skandha

Amsa-phalak

The manna points for asthma: Amsa-phalak, and Skandha.

Apply a small amount of warm Mahagenesh oil or sesame oil and finger pressure to the marma points known as Amsa-phalak and Skandha.

IMPORTANT PRECAUTIONS FOR ASTHMA

Asthma can be a life-threatening disease. Call your physician if the attack causes severe shortness of breath, if there is a bad sore throat and difficulty swallowing, or if a child is wheezing and drooling heavily. You should also consult a physician if this attack seems different from past experiences, if a child under two years of age is wheezing, or if it is uncomfortable to walk around the house or talk because of shortness of breath.

AYURVEDA

BACK AND NECK PROBLEMS

Backache is one of the most common complaints of modern civilization-80 percent of American adults suffer from back pain at some point in their lives, and it is the leading cause of worker disability. It is also one of the most difficult and frustrating conditions to treat using the tools of standard Western medicine—painkillers, muscle relaxants, antidepressants, and surgery.

Your "backbone" or spine consists of vertebrae stacked one on top of the other, ending with the sacrum (five vertebrae that fuse together during childhood) and then the coccyx (three or four small vertebrae that fuse during our twenties). In between the vertebrae are spongy disks running through the column of vertebrae that cushion the vertebral surfaces and allow the back to bend without injuring the spinal cord. Surrounding the spinal column are muscles, ligaments, and nerves, all in a complex interrelated pattern that works together to support most of your body weight while allowing you to move freely.

Most people who suffer from backaches never pinpoint the exact cause. It may be a specific injury due to overexertion or sudden movement; or it could be a lifelong posture problem finally catching up with you; or it might occur after staying in an unusual or uncomfortable position for a prolonged period of time. Often a muscle strain is involved. Ligaments along the spine and muscles in the abdomen and lower back keep the back in balance. When these muscles are weak, they can't support the torso properly. As a result they can overstretch and then strongly contract, giving us a painful muscle spasm. Being out of shape is part of the problem, and being overweight compounds the precarious situation. Ligaments (tough bands that attach bones to nearby bones) can become overstretched due to years of poor posture, putting more strain on the muscles and allowing joints to wear out, both of which can add to back problems. Emotions influence your muscles and back as well. Back complaints can even be "solutions" to hidden social and emotional conflicts or misunderstandings.

THE A-Z GUIDE

AYURVEDIC SELF-CARE

Ayurvedic practices and remedies can prevent back pain and speed healing of acute back pain due to injury. To prevent problems, follow the appropriate Daily Lifestyle Regimen for your dosha, making a strong effort to practice yoga regularly and deep breathing and alternate-nostril breathing daily. Get adequate rest—be in bed by ten P.M. and up by six A.M. If you have a sedentary job or life, sit less often—sitting puts a strain on your lower back. Change positions as often as possible. Lie down to read, stand to talk on the phone, and shift positions and take frequent breaks (about every hour) to move your back. Spending long hours standing also stresses the back. Use a back support when sitting, such as a "lumbar roll" or pillow, or a rolled-up towel taped securely to the chair back. Lose weight if you are overweight. Learn the proper way to use your back, especially when lifting heavy objects: Bend from the knees, not from the waist, and use your thigh muscles, not your back muscles. Avoid lifting until your back is healed.

If you are having back pain, apply wet heat to ease the pain. Never use dry heat directly on the skin, as it can dehydrate the tissues. You may need to rest the injury for a day or two, but prolonged bed rest is not advisable. Other healing systems can contribute to the healing process, such as acupuncture, chiropractic, osteopathy, massage, and physical therapy. A physical therapist, chiropractor, or osteopath can teach you how to move, stand, sit, sleep, bend, turn, and reach properly to reduce the stress on your back and help forestall future problems. There are also videotapes and "back schools" or "back clinics" that teach good body mechanics.

In addition the following Ayurvedic remedies will help heal and/or minimize back problems.

HERBAL REMEDIES

- Take 1/2 teaspoon triphala mixed with 1/2 cup warm water twice a day.

AYURVEDA

- Combine 1/4 teaspoon yogaraj guggulu and 1/8 teaspoon ashwaghanda (Withania somnifera) for 1 week; rest for 3 weeks, and then repeat for 1 week.

- Drink 6 ounces each of beet, cucumber, and parsley juice.

FIVE-SENSE THERAPIES

- Taste: Foods, spices, and herbs should be predominantly sweet, sour, and salty; these tastes are found in the winter churna.

- Smell: Use essential oils with sweet or warm aromas, particularly lavender, jasmine, clove, camphor, and wintergreen.

- Sight: Indigo, green, and red are the colors most frequently recommended for easing back pain.

- Hearing: Listen to the raga composed for the time during which you are experiencing pain.

- Touch: Daily oil massage (abhyanga) generally soothes back pain and prevents its recurrence.

IMPORTANT PRECAUTIONS FOR BACK AND NECK PROBLEMS

Seek medical attention if the back pain is accompanied by fever, if you have trouble with either your bowels or your bladder, your urine smells unusual or has blood in it, or you have difficulty moving or feeling your legs. Back pain can be an indication of serious health problems such as arthritis, kidney disease, or cancer. Recurrent back pain or pain that doesn't improve within one week of Ayurvedic treatment should also be evaluated professionally.

THE A-Z GUIDE

BAD BREATH

Bad breath is often blamed on something you ate or drank, such as garlic or onions, or on cigarette smoking. While these do create odors, and may be covered up with mints and such, Ayurveda considers chronic bad breath to be a digestive disorder. This pitta disorder is treated by restoring the digestive fire in the belly and the digestive juices of the mouth.

Also see Indigestion.

AYURVEDIC SELF-CARE

Follow the appropriate Daily Lifestyle Regimen for your dosha in order to set the foundation for improved digestion; it is important to eat your food when it is hot. The yoga position called Lion Pose is also recommended.

HERBAL REMEDIES

Choose one of the following:

- A simple remedy for bad breath is to chew on 1 or 2 whole cloves every day.

- Combine 1/3 teaspoon each of ajwan (celery seed), cumin, and fennel; take with 1/2 cup warm water three times a day.

- Add 1/2 teaspoon each of triphala and trikatu to 1 cup warm water; take three times a day.

- Mix 1/4 teaspoon of fresh grated ginger with a pinch of salt and eat this three times a day for strong bad breath, or once a day for chronic mild bad breath.

AYURVEDA

FIVE-SENSE THERAPIES

- Taste: Foods, herbs, and spices that are sweet, bitter, and astringent are recommended, so use the summer churna daily.

- Smell: Use essential oils with warm, spicy smells such as camphor, eucalyptus, fennel, and cinnamon.

- Sight: The color green is said to counteract bad breath.

- Hearing: Listen to the midmorning raga between the hours of ten A.M. and one P.M.

- Touch: Do a facial massage with Mahaganesh oil.

IMPORTANT PRECAUTIONS FOR BAD BREATH

Bad breath can indicate a serious digestive disorder; if this condition persists, consult a physician.

BLADDER INFECTIONS (CYSTITIS)

Bladder infections can occur in anyone—men, women, and children. However, women are affected most often, and between 10 and 15 percent of all women experience at least one bout of cystitis at some point in their lives. Although you may have an infection without noticeable symptoms, most people do suffer from at least one of the following telltale signs: burning sensation during urination, a strong urge to urinate even when little urine is passed, frequent urination (often of small amounts), a cramping feeling, and itching. Some people also have

THE A-Z GUIDE

cloudy or blood-tinged urine, lower abdominal or back pain, fever, nausea, vomiting, chills, and a general malaise.

As with all infections, cystitis results from the combination of the person's weakened resistance to infection and the presence of "germs," in this case bacteria. In women bacteria from the anus don't have far to go to reach the urethra (the tube leading from the bladder to the outside of the body). Women's urethras are only one-half inch long (compared with men's, which are several inches long and located some distance from the anus), so bacteria have only a short trip to the bladder. If the area has been irritated, for example by sex, bike riding, or the inflammation caused by a vaginal infection, a woman's ability to resist a bladder infection may be weakened.

Ayurveda recognizes differences in cystitis among the doshas. Vata-type cystitis is chronic, bothersome, and tends to come and go. The kapha type is characterized by excess mucus production. Cystitis due to a pitta imbalance causes severe burning in the bladder.

Cystitis may progress to the kidneys or bloodstream, potentially serious conditions, so it should be diagnosed initially by a health professional and monitored if symptoms are severe, prolonged, or recurrent. Antibiotics may rid the body of the current crop of bacteria but will not strengthen the body to resist future infections.

AYURVEDIC SELF-CARE

Follow the appropriate Daily Lifestyle Regimen for your dosha, with kaphas avoiding mucus-producing dairy products and pittas avoiding spices, nightshade vegetables, and alcohol. Pittas may also benefit from drinking cranberry or pomegranate juice. In addition women can prevent future occurrences of cystitis by wiping from front to back after a bowel movement and changing sanitary napkins and tampons frequently during their periods. Avoid products and practices that could irritate delicate urogenital tissues, such as deodorant products, tight clothing, and caffeine. Irritation may occur from an improperly fitted diaphragm, so check the size with your health professional; if you suspect spermicidal foams and jellies may be causing an irritation, try changing brands. You may also use the following remedies during a bout of cystitis.

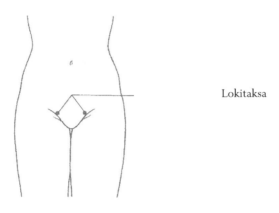

Lokitaksa

The marma points for cystitis: Lohitaksa.

Choose one of the following:

- Mix 1 to 2 teaspoons shilajit (Asphaltum) in 1/2 cup warm water and drink once or twice a day.

- Mix 1/2 teaspoon each punarnava (Boerrhavia cliffusa) and triphala in 1/2 cup warm water.

FIVE-SENSE THERAPIES

- Taste: Favor foods, herbs, and spices that are sweet, bitter, and astringent; these flavors are found in the spring churna. Kaphas especially benefit from pungent, astringent spices, such as trikatu.

- Smell: Sweet, warm smells, such as cinnamon, fennel, cloves, and sandalwood, are soothing to the bladder.

- Sight: Use lemon-yellow color therapy.

- Hearing: Listen to the late-afternoon raga between the hours of four and seven P.M.

- Touch: Apply a drop of warm sesame oil and finger pressure to the marma points called Lohitaksa.

IMPORTANT PRECAUTIONS FOR BLADDER INFECTIONS

Seek medical care if: there is pain in the kidneys; blood in the urine; headache; fever; chills; vomiting; or nausea. People with diabetes, high blood pressure, kidney disease, or recurrent cystitis should also consult a health practitioner, as should parents of children who have symptoms of urinary tract infection.

BRONCHITIS

Acute or chronic bronchitis is an inflammation of the mucous membranes of your bronchi, airways that connect the windpipe (trachea) and lungs. It is characterized by a persistent cough that often produces considerable amounts of phlegm. Acute bronchitis is usually a bacterial infection that follows a virus (such as a cold or flu); chronic bronchitis is most common in smokers and those who live in areas where the air is polluted.

Ayurveda considers the lungs to be the principal home of kapha, the earth and water dosha. Therefore most disorders of the lungs are due to a kapha imbalance and occur in people predominantly in this dosha. Accumulation of mucus indicates a low digestive fire, so Ayurvedic treatment focuses on strengthening the agni.

AYURVEDA

AYURVEDIC SELF-CARE

Follow the appropriate Daily Lifestyle Regimen for your dosha, making sure to include alternate-nostril breathing (pranayama).

HERBAL REMEDIES

Use one of the following remedies:

- For kapha: Add 1/2 teaspoon each elecampane, cinnamon, and fresh grated ginger, 1/3 teaspoon cardamom, 1 teaspoon jaggery (brown sugar), and 1 pinch cloves to 1 cup hot water and drink as a tea as often as needed.

- For vata: Add 1/2 teaspoon each elecampane, ashwaghanda, triphala, and freshly grated ginger to 1 cup hot water and drink as a tea, as needed.

- For pitta: Add 1/2 teaspoon each elecampane, burdock root, and fresh grated ginger to 1 cup hot milk and drink as often as needed.

FIVE-SENSE THERAPIES

- Taste: Use bitter, pungent, and astringent foods, herbs, and spices in your cooking and for making tea. Sprinkle the spring churna on your food every day.

- Smell: Warm, spicy aromas such as cloves, ginger, and calamus help relieve symptoms of bronchitis.

- Sight: Use the colors red, green, and orange.

- Hearing: Listen to the sunset raga between the hours of seven and ten P.M.

- Touch: Apply warm castor oil to the chest and cover with a warm compress.

IMPORTANT PRECAUTIONS FOR BRONCHITIS

Seek medical care if: there is rapid breathing; wheezing; difficulty breathing; high fever; extreme weakness; or if symptoms don't improve with Ayurvedic care within 2 days.

CELLULITE

Cellulite—that infuriating lumpiness that can occur anywhere you have fat deposits, but most commonly around the hips and thighs—is considered to be a kapha disorder. The fat cell's main job is to store energy until it is needed and then break it down and release it. But when the digestive fire is low for a long time, the fat cell accumulates kapha and gets clogged. Fat cells then keep expanding to their limits and then divide to form new cells. The bloated extra cells press against the network of collagen under the skin, resulting in the familiar cottage-cheese look. Even if you exercise and lose weight, the cellulite can remain, because the kapha energy is still stuck and the fat in the cells can't break down.

Also see Weight Problems.

AYURVEDIC SELF-CARE

Follow the appropriate Daily Lifestyle Regimen for your dosha, making sure you get enough exercise and do yoga daily.

HERBAL REMEDIES

The following internal remedy will help reduce cellulite:

- Drink one cup of hot water with 1 teaspoon of freshly grated ginger three times a day.

You may also use one or both of the following local treatments:

- Make a paste of 1 part vacha (calamus), 2 parts guggulu, and 1/4 part chitrak (Plumbago zeylonica); apply to the area with cellulite and leave in place for 1 hour before taking a warm shower.

- Massage the cellulite areas with herbal medicated oils. Use Neem oil upon arising every day; do not wash off the oil.

FIVE-SENSE THERAPIES

- Taste: Emphasize bitter, pungent, and astringent foods, spices, and herbs; these taste are found in the spring chuma.

- Sight: Favor red and orange color therapy.

- Hearing: Listen to the sunset raga between the hours of seven and ten P.M. and the midmorning raga between ten A.M. and one P.M.

- Touch: Massage the area of cellulite daily, using a silk glove and then sesame oil.

CHOLESTEROL, HIGH

Cholesterol is a normal part of your body tissues, particularly found in the blood, brain tissue, liver, kidneys, adrenal glands, and the covers around nerve fibers. Some cholesterol is needed by your body to maintain good health and body function, since it is used to form vitamin D and hormones, including the sex hormones, and to help build cell walls. However, high cholesterol in the blood has been linked with

THE A-Z GUIDE

cholesterol deposits in the blood vessels (atherosclerosis), which may in turn increase some people's risk of heart disease and stroke.

In Ayurveda high cholesterol is seen primarily as a pitta disorder. Pitta is responsible for assimilation of food and all experiences; it creates the red blood cells and controls the system of veins that carries blood to the heart. If food isn't digested and assimilated and the blood vessels aren't properly maintained, the channels of the heart become clogged.

AYURVEDIC SELF-CARE

Following the appropriate Daily Lifestyle Regimen for your dosha over the long term is the most important step you can take in controlling high cholesterol and its effects. Many studies show that exercise and a diet low in fat and high in fresh vegetables and fruits and whole grains can help lower elevated blood cholesterol. Food combinations that are said to raise cholesterol are melons with grains, eggs with milk, and milk with bananas.

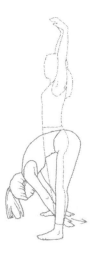

Swinging While Standing: Stand with feet 2 to 3 feet apart. Bring your arms overhead, arms straight and wrists relaxed. Bend from the hips and swing your upper body downward so that your

AYURVEDA

arms go in and out of the space between your legs five times, inhaling on each upward swing and exhaling on each downward swing. Return to the standing position with arms overhead, and then repeat up to ten times. (Note: Do not do this posture if you have vertigo or high blood pressure.)

Studies by Dr. Dean Ornish proved that a program of yoga, stress reduction, and low-fat vegetarian diet can actually reverse clogged arteries. The yoga movement swinging while standing is particularly useful for relieving this condition because it stimulates the circulation. In addition meditation has been shown to lower levels of cholesterol, according to studies done by researchers in Israel. A study done in the United States compared meditators with nonmeditators and found that people who meditated had 87.3 percent fewer admissions to the hospital for heart disease—a much greater effect than seen with any cholesterol-lowering drug available.

HERBAL REMEDIES

The general treatment for lowering cholesterol is to mix 1 teaspoon triphala in 1 cup warm water and drink at bedtime. Or you may choose one of the following to use every day until your cholesterol is lowered sufficiently:

- For vata: Add 1/2 teaspoon each arjuna (Terminalia arjuna) and haritaki (Terminalia chebula) to 1 teaspoon ghee and take every day in the morning.

- For kapha: Add 1/2 teaspoon each arjuna (Terminalia arjuna), kukti, garlic, onion, and yogaraj guggulu to 1 cup copper water; drink twice a day.

- For pitta: Take 1/2 teaspoon each arjuna (Terminalia arjuna), guduchi (Tinospora cordifolia), and manjishta (Rubia cordifolium) in 1 cup of water after lunch and dinner.

THE A-Z GUIDE

FIVE-SENSE THERAPIES

- Taste: Choose bitter, pungent, and astringent foods, herbs, and spices. Use a little spring churna on your food every day.

- Smell: Aromatherapy with warm aromas helps lower cholesterol.

- Sight: Favor the colors orange and yellow-green.

- Hearing: Listen to the midmorning raga between the hours of ten A.M. and one P.M.

- Touch: Since massage is generally relaxing and high cholesterol is linked with stress, practice relaxing abhyanga daily.

IMPORTANT PRECAUTIONS FOR HIGH CHOLESTEROL

If you have high cholesterol, it is important to be monitored by a physician.

COATED TONGUE

A whitish tongue is considered a sign of kapha imbalance and indicates accumulation of ama, undigested particles that create toxins. When the coating is at the back of the tongue only, it indicates accumulation in the large intestine; a coating in the middle of the tongue indicates accumulation in the stomach and small intestine. A white coating over the entire tongue signals toxins in the stomach, small intestine, and large intestine.

Also see Indigestion.

AYURVEDA

AYURVEDIC SELF-CARE

If your tongue is coated, following the appropriate Daily Lifestyle Regimen for your dosha should rebalance your system and clear up this condition and prevent it in the future. Be sure to scrape your tongue clean every day; gargling with sesame oil will also help. You may also try the following specific remedies to increase agni, your digestive fire.

- Combine 1/4 teaspoon trikatu and 1/2 teaspoon triphala with warm water and drink every morning for up to one month, or until the coating disappears.

- Do the Ten-Day Ginger Treatment at the beginning of every month.

- Dissolve 2 large pieces of rock candy in 1/2 cup warm water, then add 1/4 teaspoon cinnamon and a pinch of cardamom. Mix well and inhale five drops in each nostril daily.

FIVE-SENSE THERAPIES

- Taste: Bitter, pungent, and astringent foods, herbs, and spices help diminish the coating. Use the spring churna faithfully every day.

- Smell: Use essential oils with warm, spicy aromas such as camphor, eucalyptus, fennel, and cinnamon.

- Sight: Red-orange color therapy aids the digestive fire.

- Hearing: Listen to the midmorning raga between the hours of ten A.M. and one P.M. and the late-afternoon raga between four and seven P.M.

THE A-Z GUIDE

COLDS AND FLU

It's not called the "common" cold for nothing—at some point just about everyone gets one, and many people get more than one cold each year. From the Ayurvedic perspective colds are the result of an accumulation of kapha, and winter is the time when kapha accumulates most. Such an imbalance may be due to too much sleep, inactivity or forced over activity, or eating too many mucus-producing foods, such as dairy products.

Colds are usually quite benign and only require rest, a light diet, and time. However, sometimes cold symptoms can be severe enough to make you truly miserable, or may drag on for days and days. In some individuals, such as infants and young children, the elderly, and those who are immune deficient, colds can lead to more serious problems, such as secondary bacterial infections. In these people Ayurvedic medicines can help—not by suppressing sniffles, a runny nose, sneezes, a fever, sore throat, or cough but by adding support to your body's efforts to rid itself of the viral infection. Using conventional drugs to suppress cold symptoms prolongs the illness and risks drug side effects.

Flu, or influenza, is a viral infection that is sometimes confused with a cold. Both affect the upper respiratory system, but the flu is generally caused by different types of viruses that make you feel sicker than a typical cold virus does. Colds and flu share some symptoms—runny or stuffy nose, sneezing, sore throat, and cough—but flu generally also inflicts a high fever, fatigue, and a weak, ache-all-over feeling.

AYURVEDIC SELF-CARE

Make sure you take time out to rest during a cold or flu. This doesn't necessarily mean bed rest, but do take it easy so that you don't tax your reserves of energy, which could be better put to use fighting the infection. Yoga, such as a few Sun Salutations and the Lion Pose and Thunderbolt Pose, is recommended. Drink plenty of fluids to help keep mucus flowing and to replace fluid lost through sweating.

AYURVEDA

Hot, bland liquids may be particularly comforting and help to loosen phlegm. Blow your nose rather than sniffling and swallowing the mucus; cough up phlegm frequently. Nasaya (nasal-passage lubrication) is also recommended: Sniff a little ghee with 1/8 teaspoon fresh grated ginger added to clear up mucus. Avoid extreme heat, such as steam baths and saunas, and extreme cold as well. Keep the air moist with a humidifier or vaporizer; or inhale steam from a bowl of hot water (make a hood by draping a towel over your head) to further loosen mucus and make breathing easier. Eat a light diet of bland, well-cooked food.

There are a large number of Ayurvedic remedies useful for cold and flu symptoms. The most commonly used are listed below. If the infection you are treating is accompanied by other symptoms, refer to other sections such as Fever, Coughs, and Sore Throats.

HERBAL REMEDIES

Use one or more of the following:

- Add 1/2 teaspoon pippali (long pepper) to 1 cup warm water and drink as needed.

- Combine 4 parts sesame oil with 1 part black mustard seed to make mustard oil; take 1 teaspoon of this plus 1 teaspoon of jaggery (brown sugar) orally, as needed.

- For colds or flu with congestion, cough, and runny nose: Add 1/4 teaspoon fresh grated ginger and 1/2 teaspoon cinnamon to 1 cup hot water; drink this two or three times a day.

- For colds and flu with cough and congestion: Add 1 pinch cloves, 1/2 teaspoon fresh grated ginger, and 1 teaspoon honey to 1 cup hot water; drink this two or three times a day.

THE A-Z GUIDE

- For colds or flu with congestion and fever: Add 1/3 teaspoon each cumin, coriander, and fennel to 1 cup hot water; drink this three times a day.

- For children: Add 1 pinch each pippali (long pepper), black pepper, fresh grated ginger, and sitopaladi to 1 cup warm to hot water; drink this three times a day.

FIVE-SENSE THERAPIES

- Taste: Emphasize foods that are sweet, sour, and salty, and use the winter churna, which also provides these tastes.

- Smell: Use essential oils with warm, spicy aromas such as eucalyptus, camphor, and cloves.

- Sight: Blue and green are particularly healing for colds or flu.

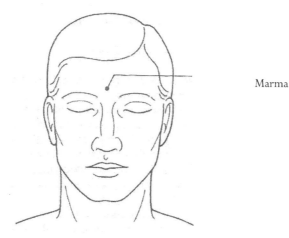

Marma

The marma point for colds and flu: Ajna.

- Hearing: Listen to the late-afternoon raga between the hours of one and four P.M. and the sunset raga between seven and ten P.M.

- Touch: Apply one drop of warm sesame oil and finger pressure to the marma points known as Pleeha and Ajna.

IMPORTANT PRECAUTIONS FOR COLDS AND FLU

Seek medical care if symptoms are unusually severe, or if there is: severe difficulty breathing or shortness of breath; chest pain; convulsions; delirium; high fever; extreme weakness; a stiff neck; wheezing; severe headache; or sudden, unexpected vomiting. Also consult your Ayurvedic practitioner if you get upper respiratory infections frequently or if they are severe and long lasting.

CONFUSION, POOR CONCENTRATION, AND FORGETFULNESS

Although confusion, poor concentration, and forgetfulness are equated with getting older, these annoying conditions can happen to anyone at any age. Midsentence you completely lose your train of thought; you meet someone for the first time and immediately forget his or her name; having just entered a room, you can't for the life of you figure out why you went there; balancing your checkbook is a thankless challenge.

Often a vata imbalance is at the root; an Ayurvedic practitioner would say the energy flow from the diaphragm is moving upward to the brain. It's easy to see why vata could become aggravated, because today we are bombarded with stimulation to the point of being overstimulated. In an effort to stay caught up, many people are simply trying to do too much and stuff too many pieces of information into their gray matter. Although studies show that an appropriate amount of stimulation causes new brain

THE A-Z GUIDE

cells to grow, too much causes stress and appears to cause the brain to shut down and possibly deteriorate.

Although sometimes an emergency sharpens the mind, poor concentration very often accompanies anxiety. You may be so worried you "can't think." Another possibility is that your brain may not be getting enough oxygen or nutrients. These symptoms may also occur because of food allergies or sensitivities, poor sleep patterns, or depression. (Also see Insomnia and Depression.) Many commonly prescribed drugs and nonprescription drugs affect the concentration as well. If you find you're not the brilliant, clear-thinking genius you want to be, the following natural approaches offer safe ways to help you clear your muddled mind.

AYURVEDIC SELF-CARE

As you follow the appropriate Daily Lifestyle Regimen to balance your doshas, you may be able to quiet your overly busy, confused mind through relaxation and meditation. Meditation helps disperse thoughts, leaving a clean slate for clearer thinking. And yoga is wonderful for clearing and refreshing the mind. There are also many methods and tricks used to improve memory and concentration. Jogging your memory is like jogging your body—you need to exercise it in order to develop it fully.

So if you're bored and understimulated, read new books, get out and meet new people; attend lectures, museums, and group discussions. But remember, too much stimulation is stressful, so if you fall into this category, think of ways you can streamline your life. Just as you can over exercise your body, so you can overtax your brain; give both the rest they need so that they can recharge.

AYURVEDA

HERBAL REMEDIES

Combine 1/4 teaspoon jatamansi (Nordostachys jatamansi) and 1/4 teaspoon each sarsaluti and trikatu with 1/2 cup warm water; drink daily.

- Add 1/2 teaspoon yogaraj guggulu 'to vata tea and drink daily.

FIVE-SENSE THERAPIES

- Taste: Favor sweet, sour, and salty tastes when choosing and preparing food and teas. The winter churna is also a good source of these tastes.

- Smell: Calamus oil is reputed to help clear and sharpen the mind.

- Sight: Blue-green color therapy freshens the mind.

- Hearing: Listen to the sunrise raga between seven and ten A.M. and the sunset raga between seven and ten P.M.

- Touch: Apply warm sesame oil and massage your forehead, ears, and the points where the back of your skull meets your neck.

IMPORTANT PRECAUTIONS FOR CONFUSION, POOR CONCENTRATION, AND FORGETFULNESS

Confusion, forgetfulness, and poor concentration can be signs of a serious brain disease, such as Alzheimer's, or other brain damage that is due to small, undetected strokes caused by high blood pressure. They can also signal the presence of a previously undiagnosed low thyroid condition (hypothyroidism) or low blood sugar (hypoglycemia). If the symptoms are new; come on suddenly; are accompanied by blurred vision, headaches, or vomiting; or seem to be getting worse, contact your physician.

THE A-Z GUIDE

CONSTIPATION

Constipation—difficult, incomplete, or infrequent bowel movements—
is one of the many side effects of too much "civilization." Contributing
factors are a diet that overemphasizes hard-to-digest foods or food
combinations. Too little exercise, too much tension and stress, or overstimulation of the nervous system, including too much TV, can cause
constipation. Sometimes travel, with its multitude of changes, also brings
temporary constipation until we adjust.

In Ayurveda constipation is often a sign of low agni or digestive fire and
an accumulation of ama. When constipated, you may feel sluggish and
bloated, and you usually have a coated tongue. This condition is usually
associated with a vata imbalance; too much air from this dosha dries out
the stool. Being "regular" means having at least one bowel movement
first thing in the morning every day, and stool should float. It is normal
for balanced pitta types to have up to three bowel movements a day.

A prolonged and noticeable change in bowel habits may be a sign of
serious disease, such as cancer or other intestinal illnesses. A tendency to
chronic constipation means the bowels and nervous system are out of
kilter and should be evaluated by a professional health care practitioner.

AYURVEDIC SELF-CARE

Constipation should respond to and be prevented by following the
appropriate Daily Lifestyle Regimen for your dosha. Watch your diet:
Eat plenty of fresh fruits, vegetables, and beans to add natural fiber. Fiber
(roughage) is not absorbed in the intestine and acts as a sponge to hold
water, creating a bulkier, softer stool, which stimulates bowel
contractions and easier, more frequent passage. Small amounts of
healthful oily foods such as ghee help lubricate the whole body, including
the digestive tract. Be sure to eat only the recommended food
combinations and avoid processed foods such as white flour and sugar, as
well as cheese and meat. Drink adequate fluids, especially plain warm or
hot water throughout the day, or fruit juice diluted with water, to work

AYURVEDA

with the fiber; sodas, coffee, and large quantities of black or orange pekoe tea are not recommended. Adding pure bran (oat or wheat) to your diet is not advised unless recommended by a nutrition specialist. It's better to eat whole grains such as oatmeal, Wheatena, and brown rice, which naturally contain bran. Exercise will stimulate your digestive organs and also help keep things moving along as they should be. Yoga will relax the nervous system and stimulate the organs; the Leg Cycling Pose and the Leg Lock Pose are particularly helpful.

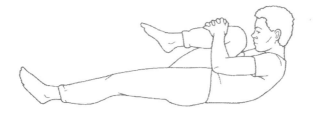

Leg Lock Pose: Lying on your back, bend one leg, bringing your thigh close to your chest. Inhale deeply as you clasp your hands around the shin, just under the knee. Exhale, and lift your head and upper chest toward the knee. Exhale as you slowly release. Repeat ten times with each leg.

If you are very uncomfortable, the specific Ayurvedic remedies recommended below will help you overcome sluggish bowels. Try to avoid taking strong laxatives, even occasionally; but if you must, use either psyllium seed (Metamucil is a well-known brand name), which is a bulk laxative; stewed prunes or prune juice; or an enema to get things moving again. But be aware it is all too easy to become dependent on these artificial means, which, like any crutch, weaken the system and do not get to the root of the problem.

HERBAL REMEDIES

- For gentle-to-moderate stimulation of movement: Take 1 teaspoon of either triphala, psyllium husks, senna, or flaxseed along with 1 cup warm to hot water at bedtime until your constipation is relieved.

THE A-Z GUIDE

- For strong stimulation of movement: Take a combination of the four above remedies or 1 teaspoon aloe vera gel at bedtime.

- For constipation with gas (flatulence): Take either 1/2 teaspoon haritaki (Terminalia chebula) or triphala, along with a pinch of salt in 1/4 cup warm water until the condition subsides.

FIVE-SENSE THERAPIES

- Taste: Emphasize foods, herbs, and spices that are sweet, sour, and salty, such as are found in the winter churna.

- Smell: Aromas that are warm and spicy, such as clove, cinnamon, lavender, and calamus, help ease constipation.

- Sight: Red and yellow color therapy may be helpful.

- Hearing: Listen to the late-afternoon raga between the hours of four and seven P.M. and the sunset raga between seven and ten P.M.

- Touch: Apply a small amount of warm sesame oil and massage the navel area daily.

IMPORTANT PRECAUTIONS FOR CONSTIPATION

Seek medical care if you have not had a bowel movement in 24 hours and you have severe or unusual pain; if the constipation has lasted more than two weeks; if your stools are consistently black, gray, or white; if your eyes or skin are yellowish (jaundiced); if you alternate constipation with diarrhea; if blood accompanies the stools; or if constipation is accompanied by very thin stools, abdominal pain, and bloating or unexplained weight loss.

AYURVEDA

COUGHS

Coughing is a reflex that acts as a defense mechanism. An irritation or obstruction in one of the breathing tubes triggers the mechanism, which creates a strong upward rush of air. This explosive movement forces the irritating or obstructing material out of the tube. Coughing also helps to aerate the lungs and reorganize the breathing mechanisms.

Coughing often accompanies viral or bacterial infections; these include colds, influenza, croup (harsh, barking cough in young children), laryngitis, bronchitis, and pneumonia. Other causes are a postnasal drip, often related to allergies—mucus from the nose drains into the breathing tubes, causing an irritating tickle. Smoking cigarettes causes continual irritation of the tubes and is the number-one cause of coughs. In addition the mind-body doesn't necessarily distinguish between a physical and an emotional or social irritant resulting in a cough.

In Ayurveda a dry cough is a sign of a vata imbalance, a cough accompanied by infection is associated with a pitta imbalance, and a "productive" cough (mucus) is due to a kapha imbalance.

AYURVEDIC SELF-CARE

Home care is similar to that for colds; see that section for details, especially if the cough is due to a cold. The yoga position known as Lion Pose is therapeutic for coughs. It's helpful to rest, drink fluids, and try to cough up any phlegm; increasing the humidity in the room thins the mucus and makes it easier to expel—this is particularly essential treatment for children with the croup. Drinking hot beverages also liquifies mucus. There are many Ayurvedic remedies used to treat coughs. The most commonly used are listed below.

Also see Colds, Fever, or Sore Throat if any of these accompany the cough.

THE A-Z GUIDE

HERBAL REMEDIES

In addition to taking 1 teaspoon triphala mixed with 1/4 cup warm water at bedtime, you may take:

- For cough with chest pain: Combine 5 parts shatavari (Asparagus racemosus), 3 parts guduchi (Tinospora cordifolia), 2 parts abhrak, and 3 parts auypatik kara

- churna; take 1/2 teaspoon of this mixture three times a day mixed with 1 cup warm water.

- For chronic cough: Mix together 1/2 teaspoon black pepper and 1 teaspoon honey; take this mixture two or three times a day.

- For a dry (vata) cough: Mix equal parts fennel powder and rock candy; chew as needed. Or make a tea by combining 1 teaspoon fennel seeds with 1 cup hot water and let steep for 20 minutes; strain, add 1 teaspoon honey and 1/2 lemon and drink as needed.

- For a productive (kapha) cough: Boil together 1/2 teaspoon turmeric powder and 1 cup milk; drink at night.

FIVE-SENSE THERAPIES

- Taste: Sweet, bitter, and astringent tastes are soothing for coughs; these tastes are found in the summer churna.

- Smell: Use essential oils with sweet, warm, spicy aromas, particularly mint, eucalyptus, camphor, and fennel.

- Sight Yellow-green or blue-green are therapeutic for coughs.

- Hearing: Listen to raga music composed for the hours when you are most uncomfortable.

AYURVEDA

- Touch: Apply warm castor oil to the chest and back,   massage in well, and cover with a warm compress.

IMPORTANT PRECAUTIONS FOR COUGHS

Seek medical care if: the cough began suddenly and violently in a child who does not have a cold and who may have swallowed a foreign object; it occurs in an infant under three months of age; rapid breathing, difficulty breathing, or wheezing accompanies the cough; it is severe and doesn't respond to home care in two days; or there is prolonged high fever or extreme weakness.

DEPRESSION

Feeling sad is a normal part of the ups and downs of life. Normal sadness is a temporary thing, and usually linked with a specific event or loss—the death of a loved one, the breakup of a marriage, being passed over for a job promotion. This is not the same as depression, which drains the pleasure out of life, leaving you feeling in pain yet numb, at the bottom of a deep black hole, with seemingly no way out or light at the end of the tunnel, your mind filled with negative thoughts.

Depression seems to be more common now than it was fifty or one hundred years ago: between ten and fourteen million Americans suffer from this frustrating, puzzling condition. Fortunately you can self-treat mild depression with Ayurveda, but it's very important to identify the underlying cause of your problem and to seek professional help for moderate or severe episodes. These triggers include the following:

- Loneliness and lack of social support as a child and as an adult
- BoredomRecent major stressful events, traumatic experiences, and grief
- Parents who suffered from depression

THE A-Z GUIDE

- Medical illnesses and medication
- Lack of sunlight
- Abuse of alcohol and other drugs

From the Ayurvedic point of view most depression is a kapha imbalance that is the culmination of vata and then pitta going out of balance. Initially the brain's electrochemistry has an erratic overreaction (vata imbalance), which triggers a loss of enzymatic activity in the metabolism (pitta imbalance). Kapha responds by trying to glue everything down, bringing about heaviness, darkness, and stagnation that the mind-body interprets as the negative message of hopelessness and depression. Sometimes depression is a pitta disorder. Allergies and the breakdown in metabolic processes they lead to can also disturb brain chemistry. This can cause dramatic mood swings, with depression as one of the consequences.

No one should go around feeling depressed just because they always have. Sometimes it goes away by itself, but why wait? Depression is a disease that has effective treatments—whether through the natural approaches suggested here, or psychotherapy, or medication, or a combination—which can make it go away sooner. Mild to moderate depression may respond to Ayurveda alone, or this approach may be used along with psychotherapy for optimum effectiveness.

Also see Mood Swings and Irritability, Fatigue, and Anxiety and Fear.

AYURVEDIC SELF-CARE

Following the appropriate Daily Lifestyle Regimen for your dosha over the long term usually helps keep you on a more even keel. You should also be aware that depression is a possible side effect of caffeine and aspartame, and of food and chemical allergy or sensitivity. Depression may also be caused by certain drugs and has been linked with cigarette smoking. Since stress is a known depressant, try to be extra good to yourself and consider exploring ways to relax daily and manage stress

AYURVEDA

better, such as meditation and yoga. Regular strenuous physical activity is the cornerstone of any effort to overcome depression. Studies show it's a superb mood elevator and stress buster in addition to its many other health-improving benefits. We especially recommend activities that get you out into the world with other people, such as dancing and aerobics classes. The yoga positions called the Shoulder Stand and the Plow help elevate mood.

In Ayurveda it is especially important to get up before sunrise; if you arise after the kapha time of day begins, it makes you feel all the heavier, more lethargic, and more depressed. If your depression seems seasonal and is better or nonexistent during the time of the year when days are longer, you might have seasonal affective disorder (SAD).

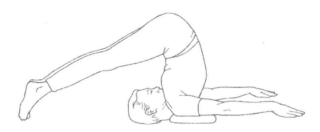

The Plow: Lie on your back with a folded towel or pillow under your shoulders, arms straight beside you, palms down. Lift your legs and torso up and over your head until your toes touch the floor. Keep your legs straight if possible. Hold this position for fifteen seconds to one minute, breathing evenly and deeply throughout. Ib come out of this pose, bend your knees and exhale as you slowly roll out the spine. (Note: Stop immediately if you feel pain—contrasted with discomfort—while entering or doing this pose.)

Particularly common in wintertime in northern climates, SAD is a form of depression due to lack of sunlight; it is treated successfully with exposure to bright artificial light that mimics natural sunlight. So if you suspect you might have a mild form of SAD, try to spend more time in sunlight—indoors and out. Consider taking winter vacations to sunny climates, sit near an open window or skylight, and replace standard fluorescent or incandescent bulbs with full-spectrum ones.

THE A-Z GUIDE

Psychosocial remedies for depression include seeing your friends, getting out and going to parties, perhaps attending or forming a support group, and a determined refusal to accept anyone's low regard for any reason. The very act of bestirring yourself to action could help chase the black clouds away.

HERBAL REMEDIES

Regardless of the type of depression you are experiencing, use all three of the following remedies:

- Combine 5 parts shatavari (Asparagus racemosus), 3 parts jatamansi (Nordostachys jatamansi), 3 parts brahmi (gotu kola), and 5 parts guduchi (Tinospora cordifolia); take 1/4 teaspoon of this mixture with 1/2 cup warm water three times a day.

- Take 1 teaspoon triphala with 1/2 cup warm water at bedtime every night.

- Inhale 3 drops of Brahmi oil into each nostril twice a day, and rub the oil on the sides of your feet at bedtime.

- In addition, use one of the following herbal combinations, depending on the type of depression you are experiencing:

- Vata depression is characterized by anxiety and hopelessness and light, dry, mobile, active behavior. Take 1/2 teaspoon each brahmi (gotu kola), vacha (calamus), and jatamansi (Nordostachys jatamansi), and 1 teaspoon shankhapushpi (Crotalatia verrucosa); take 1/4 teaspoon of this mixture with 1/2 cup warm water three times a day.

- Pitta depression makes a person feel angry and disturbed. In this case the remedy is 1/2 teaspoon shatavari

AYURVEDA

- (Asparagus racemosus) and 1/4 teaspoon guduchi (Tinospora cordifolia) combined with 1/2 cup warm water.

- Kapha depression is characterized by heaviness, dullness, and slowness. Combine 1 part each brahmi (gotu kola), trikatu, jatamansi (Nordostachys jatamansi), and licorice with 1/2 part vacha (calamus); take 1/2 teaspoon of this mixture combined with warm water three times a day until the depression begins to lift.

FIVE-SENSE REMEDIES

- Taste: Use bitter, pungent, and astringent foods, herbs, and spices. Spring churna is recommended.

- Smell: Warm aromas such as cloves, calamus, and camphor are effective aromatherapy.

- Sight: Use the color red.

- Hearing: Listen to the sunset raga between seven and ten P. M.

- Touch: Give yourself a silk glove massage daily.

IMPORTANT PRECAUTIONS FOR DEPRESSION

Depression can be a serious illness—it can affect your whole life and possibly produce thoughts of suicide. Depression has detrimental effects on your physical body, particularly the immune system, and has recently even been linked with accelerated bone loss in women. If Ayurveda hasn't helped and you are "down" for more than four months after a difficult event, such as a death in the family—or if sadness lasts more than a couple of weeks and you can't pinpoint the cause of your blues— you should seek advice, counseling, and perhaps medication from a mental health professional. Depression can be readily diagnosed and controlled by a combination of supportive counseling and medication with any one of a number of products.

The established criteria for diagnosing major depression include the presence of a depressed, irritable mood with loss of interest or pleasure in usual activities, including sex, plus at least four other of the following symptoms over a two-week period:

- Poor appetite and weight loss or increased appetite with weight gain
- Disturbed sleep (too much, too little)
- Excess physical activity or inactivity—agitation or lethargy
- Fatigue and loss of energy
- Feelings of worthlessness, self-reproach, excessive guilt
- Thoughts of or attempts at suicide
- Difficulty thinking, concentrating, or making decisions; forgetfulness

DERMATITIS/ECZEMA

Ayurveda says, "Know your skin, know your inner organs." The state of your skin reflects your inner health, particularly that of your digestive system. Hot skin indicates inner anger, whereas cold skin indicates fear or anxiety. Dermatitis and eczema are inflammatory skin conditions that indicate a severe pitta imbalance. When your digestive fire is low, ama forms, clogging the system and compromising your immunity. As a result you become sensitive to substances in your environment such as detergent, jewelry, or cosmetics. Clearing up skin disorders is an inside as well as an outside job.

AYURVEDA

AYURVEDIC SELF-CARE

If you have chronic skin problems, you need to follow a Daily Lifestyle Regimen to balance your doshas, regulate your digestive system, restore your digestive fire, cleanse and strengthen your liver, and cleanse and oil your skin and remove old skin daily (abhyanga). Stress is often a factor in skin eruptions, and therefore meditation is a cornerstone treatment for skin conditions.

You may also want to try to determine what triggers the rash so that you can eliminate it from the environment. To prevent the rash from becoming infected with bacteria or fungus, wash gently with mild soap (such as calendula soap) and water twice a day. Apply Neem oil to soothe the raw skin; wet comfrey tea compresses are particularly soothing for poison oak. Change clothes once or twice a day to keep the skin clean; or you may cover the affected areas with loose sterile gauze dressings. Keep the affected areas away from water as much as possible. You may need to reduce bathing and washing, and wear protective rubber gloves for hand washing of clothes or dishes.

Avoid strong soaps. Use gentle soaps without perfumes or chemicals sparingly. Lubricate the skin with sesame oil (vata types), coconut oil (pittas), or any light oil (kaphas). Try not to scratch, because it irritates already inflamed skin.

HERBAL REMEDIES

- The Ayurvedic remedy most commonly used to treat dermatitis and eczema is turmeric powder, applied directly to the skin three times a day. Use carefully—it will stain clothing.

- You may also mix 1/2 teaspoon vidanga (Embelia ribes), 1/2 teaspoon ghee, and 1 teaspoon honey with 1/2 cup warm water; using an eyedropper, insert 5 drops into each nostril and sniff, once or twice a day.

THE A-Z GUIDE

FIVE-SENSE THERAPIES

- Taste: Favor sweet, bitter, and astringent foods, spices, and herbs. Add a little salt and lemon flakes to the summer churna and use this to flavor your food every day.

- Smell: Sweet, bitter, and cool aromas such as jasmine, sandalwood, and mint sooth skin eruptions.

- Sight: Use blue or indigo color therapy.

- Hearing: Listen to the midmorning raga music between the hours of ten A.M. and one P.M.

- Touch: Massage with Neem oil is helpful for all three doshas; sesame oil may also be used for vata and pitta types.

IMPORTANT PRECAUTIONS FOR DERMATITIS AND ECZEMA

If you see signs, of infection such as pus and worsening inflammation, see a physician. If the acute eczema returns again and again, it is probably a chronic condition and should be treated professionally.

DIARRHEA

Transient or isolated incidents of loose bowel movements and associated symptoms are not cause for concern; they usually resolve themselves quickly. Frequent, prolonged diarrhea poses the danger of dehydration, especially in infants when it is accompanied by vomiting and sweating due to fever. Chronic diarrhea is usually due to a vata imbalance. The vata components of digestion do not work in sequence, and the ileocecal valve, located between the large and small intestines, opens and becomes spastic. This leads to pressure in the colon and forces it to give up its

AYURVEDA

contents prematurely. Although it is a vata imbalance, diarrhea manifests itself variously depending on each person's prominent dosha. Ayurvedic self-care including specific Ayurvedic remedies usually helps the digestive tract return to normal.

AYURVEDIC SELF-CARE

Home care revolves around replacing lost fluids and slow, gentle reintroduction of easily digested foods. If you experience diarrhea frequently, you need to faithfully follow the Daily Lifestyle Regimen most appropriate for balancing your dosha. During a bout of diarrhea, limit eating for up to twelve hours after the first symptoms of diarrhea appear. This prevents stimulating the digestive system, which could cause more diarrhea. Gradually introduce clear liquids to replace the water the body has lost. Water, diluted fruit juice, bouillon, and rice water (use double the usual amount of water and drain after cooking) are examples. Next introduce bland solid foods, which tend to slow down the bowels. Think "BRAT": Bananas, Rice, Applesauce, and Toast. Avoid fatty foods, hard-to-digest foods, and milk and milk products, although nonfat yogurt may be tolerated. Offer fluids often to young children, who may want only small amounts at a time.

- The mainstay of Ayurvedic treatment for acute diarrhea is 1 pinch triphala mixed with 1 teaspoon ghee, taken twice a day.

- Another commonly used general remedy is 1/2 teaspoon powdered ginger and 1 teaspoon fennel powder, mixed with 1 teaspoon ghee, taken twice a day.

- Chronic diarrhea usually responds to 1 or 2 teaspoons triphala with 1/2 cup warm water at bedtime, and roasted cumin or fennel seeds chewed after meals.

- In addition you may take 1 teaspoon ghee mixed with a pinch of one of the following:

THE A-Z GUIDE

* Rock salt—for vata imbalance characterized by pain, cramping, passing of gas, and frequent movements without passing much stool; diarrhea may alternate with constipation

* Nutmeg—for pitta imbalance characterized by stool that is yellow, smells bad, is hot, and is accompanied by a burning sensation in the rectal area

* Ginger—for kapha imbalance characterized by whitish stools that may contain phlegm or mucus and are accompanied by lethargy and heaviness.

FIVE-SENSE THERAPIES

- Taste: Emphasize sweet, sour, and salty tastes, which can be found in the winter churna.

- Smell: Sweet, warm aromas work best for diarrhea.

- Sight: Use the color green for color therapy.

- Hearing: Listen to the late-afternoon raga between the hours of four and seven P.M.

- Touch: Apply a drop of warm sesame oil and finger pressure to the marma points known as Kukundara. You may also massage warm castor oil over the area of cramping.

AYURVEDA

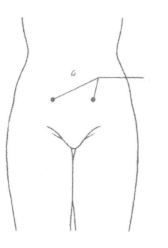

Kukundara

The marma points for diarrhea: Kukundara.

IMPORTANT PRECAUTIONS FOR DIARRHEA

Medical care should be sought if the diarrhea continues for 3 days. Watch for signs of dehydration, especially in infants and young children; this requires professional evaluation and can occur in twelve to twenty-four hours in adults and eight to twelve hours in children. A professional should also be consulted if: the stools are black or bloody; there is severe abdominal pain; or there is unusual vaginal bleeding or persistent pain in women of childbearing age.

EARACHES

Earaches can happen at any age, but most often occur in children. The average child experiences at least one ear infection by age six, and some children are plagued by a series of them. Ayurveda believes that recurrent earaches are due to faulty digestive and elimination systems,

THE A-Z GUIDE

which lead to toxic accumulation of ama and a weakening of the immune system. In children and adult ear infections come in two varieties:

Otitis media is an infection of the middle ear, the space behind the eardrum. Colds and allergies often lay the groundwork for middle-ear infections by narrowing the eustachian tube that leads from the middle ear to the nasal passages. The ear fluids that normally drain through the tube into the throat accumulate in this space, causing blockage and a comfortable environment for bacteria to grow in. Young children are particularly vulnerable because their tubes are so small and short. In children symptoms are ear pain, fever, crying and fussiness, pulling the ears, restless sleep, and temporary hearing loss. The eardrum may rupture and allow a discharge to flow out. The rupture usually heals completely in a few weeks with no permanent consequences. Ayurvedic remedies provide a safe, effective way of avoiding antibiotics, which can weaken defenses and encourage further ear infections.

Otitis externa is a skin infection of the ear canal that leads from the outer ear in toward the eardrum. Also related to bacteria, this is a shallow infection and less serious than otitis media. "Swimmer's ear," common in summer and among year-round serious swimmers, is a form of otitis externa. Symptoms are redness, inflammation, itchiness, and pain when the outer ear is moved, such as occurs when the earlobe is tugged.

AYURVEDIC SELF-CARE

In curing and preventing earache, the twin goals of Ayurveda are to eliminate toxins by cleaning the system and strengthening the digestive system so that toxins don't accumulate in the first place. Following the Daily Lifestyle Regimen for balancing your doshas and the cleansing and agni-strengthening practices should go a long way toward strengthening the immune system, and aid in the recovery from ear infection.

When acute ear pain strikes, as with any infection, rest helps the healing process. Consuming plenty of fluids helps keep secretions fluid and replaces water lost through perspiration. Avoid all dairy and wheat products during an acute infection. Moist heat, such as a hot towel or washcloth or a hot-water bottle, may soothe pain. Some people find that cold relieves pain. Flush out packed-in wax with a syringe filled with warm water or hydrogen peroxide diluted with four parts water, but avoid inserting objects to clean out ears. It's also helpful to learn to evaluate and diagnose ear infections. Ask your health care professional to show you how to use an otoscope (available at pharmacies) to examine the ears of family members.

HERBAL REMEDIES

- As soon as symptoms appear, begin the basic approach of cleaning the colon and detoxifying the system by using triphala, the mild and safe yet effective Ayurvedic remedy. Mix together 1 pinch triphala and 1/2 cup blackberry or blueberry juice; drink this twice on each of the first two days of symptoms, then once on the third day. Insert 2 drops each of garlic and mullein oil (available at health food stores), every 2 hours until the pain is soothed.

FIVE-SENSE THERAPIES

- Taste: Emphasize sweet, bitter, and astringent tastes; these are easily obtained from the summer churna and from pitta foods.

- Smell: Use aromatherapy with warm, spicy aromas such as camphor, eucalyptus, and mint.

- Sight: Blue or yellow-green color therapy is helpful.

- Hearing: Listen to the raga appropriate to the time of day, particularly during the sunset (seven to ten P.M.) and late afternoon (four to seven P.M.).

- Touch: Apply warm castor oil compresses on the ear and area where the jawbone meets the ear. To make the compress, fold a washcloth twice lengthwise and, holding on to the ends, dip the center into hot water. Twist to squeeze out excess water; apply 1 tablespoon castor oil to the center portion and apply to the ear. As it loses its heat, redip the cloth and reapply. You may also apply a drop of Brahmi oil to both ears, on the marma point, and apply firm pressure.

IMPORTANT PRECAUTIONS FOR EARACHES

Medical care should be sought if Ayurvedic remedies fail to improve an earache within 24 hours in a young child, or in 2 to 3 days in an older child or adult. Get medical care if there is: extreme weakness, severe pain, or stiff neck; any swelling, redness, or pain behind the ear; fever accompanied by a profuse ear discharge; hearing loss that extends beyond 2 weeks. Have the ear examined by your health care practitioner three weeks after successful Ayurvedic treatment to make sure the healing is complete.

ELECTRONIC POLLUTION

Electronic pollution is becoming an increasing problem in modern society. Common electronic devices such as TVs, microwave ovens, computers, and cellular phones (as well as power lines and transformers) bathe everyone with their electromagnetic energy fields. Many scientists believe that this poses an insidious health problem and cite evidence that suggests that electronic pollution may increase risk of cancer and reproductive problems, and affect the immune system and behavior. How this occurs eludes scientists, but some research shows that certain types of electromagnetic radiation disrupt the cues that keep our biological cycles properly timed.

According to Ayurveda, too much exposure to computers, television, and cellular phones affects the prana, the vital force that pulses through your mind-body. Prana is the bioenergetic magnetic field of the brain. It

AYURVEDA

is the director of the mind, senses, intellect, and reasoning; its circuitry relays stimuli from the brain directly to the heart.

If not overexposed, the brain adapts and can "digest" this energy. But overexposure inundates the brain and hypothalamus, jamming them with information, locking them into an overstimulated state. Immediate symptoms are eyestrain, headache, fatigue, and a disoriented flu-like feeling. If you've noticed these symptoms after, for example, spending hours and hours in front of a computer, you may have suffered from a vata imbalance due to electronic pollution. Electronic smog is impossible to avoid completely, but you can balance your doshas so that you are better able to withstand it. Ayurveda also offers remedies for when overexposure does occur.

AYURVEDIC SELF-CARE

Follow the Daily Lifestyle Regimen that will balance your doshas and strengthen your resistance to electromagnetic exposure. In addition try to minimize your exposure as much as possible. Electric-blanket manufacturers have recently changed their design so as to minimize electromagnetic fields; but if you have an old one, you should use it only on occasion. When watching TV or using a computer, sit as far away as possible. Take frequent breaks and buy a radiation shield for your computer screen. Ask yourself if you really need to use your cell phone or your microwave oven. If you notice symptoms of overexposure, use the following remedies.

HERBAL REMEDIES

- Drink a cup of warm milk to which you have added a pinch of saffron.

- Drink a cup of vata tea to which you have added 1/2 teaspoon jatamansi (Nordostachys jatamansi) and 1/4 teaspoon saraswati.

THE A-Z GUIDE

FIVE-SENSE THERAPIES

- Taste: Eat foods, herbs, and spices that are predominantly sweet, sour, and salty in taste. The winter churna is a good source for these tastes.

- Smell: Inhale aromas that are sweet and warm to counteract electronic pollution; for example, orange, basil, and jasmine.

- Sight: Use green for color therapy.

- Hearing: Listen to the raga appropriate to the time that you use electronic devices such as computers.

- Touch: Daily abhyanga will help calm vata.

IMPORTANT PRECAUTIONS FOR ELECTRONIC POLLUTION

Long-term habitual exposure to electromagnetic fields such as that which occurs in particular occupations has been found by researchers to cause certain health disorders. Know the degree of your exposure and the risks; if possible, avoid exposure, and wear protective clothing if you are exposed. Be sure to see your doctor if you notice signs of tinnitus (ringing in the ears), visual disturbances, nausea, or headache.

EMOTIONAL INERTIA OR OBSESSION

Emotional inertia occurs when you get stuck in an emotional state that refuses to dissolve. Being trapped in a negative message, you seem to have a million and one good reasons for not moving on to a more productive thought process. Low self-esteem is a classic case in point: "I'm no good. I'll never be able to do that."

AYURVEDA

The neurotransmitters that your brain releases direct your senses to sleep, eat, feel, react, and be human. When vata becomes imbalanced, these neurojuices are undernourished emotionally or physically traumatized—they break down. This leads to obsessing because the brain cannot produce the next set of neurotransmitters to finish the thought process and start a new one.

AYURVEDIC SELF-CARE

Follow the appropriate Daily Lifestyle Regimen to balance your doshas. The series of yoga movements called Sun Salutation is particularly useful for relieving this condition.

HERBAL REMEDIES

- Combine 1 part jatamansi (Nordostachys jatamansi) and 2 parts saraswati; add 1 part shatavari (Asparagus racemosus) (for women) or. 1 part ashwaghanda (Withania somnifera) (for men); take up to 1/2 teaspoon mixed with 1 cup warm milk or water, two or three times a day.

- Combine 2 parts gotu kola and 1 part arjun (Tenninalia arjuna); take 1 teaspoon mixed with warm milk or water twice a day.

FIVE-SENSE THERAPIES

- Taste: Emphasize foods, herbs, and spices that are sweet, sour, and salty. These flavors predominate in the winter churna.

- Smell: Use essential oils that have sweet and warm smells, such as sage, basil, orange, and rose.

- Sight: Green color therapy helps dislodge stuck thought patterns.

THE A-Z GUIDE

- Hearing: Listen to the midday raga between the hours of one and four P.M.

- Touch: Do facial massage daily using warm sesame oil   and applying finger pressure to the marma points.

IMPORTANT PRECAUTIONS FOR EMOTIONAL INERTIA

If Ayurveda doesn't help you get past your emotional inertia, consult a physician.

FATIGUE

Although low energy and fatigue are often viewed as inevitable signs of aging, a healthy body at any age supports a healthy, active mind. Fatigue and low energy are often signs of our bodies crying out for help.

In Ayurveda fatigue is a tridoshic disorder; that is, it involves all three doshas. First, vata becomes imbalanced, then the pitta fire loses its strength, and kapha becomes heavier and heavier as it tries to ground the windy vata. If the windy vata becomes a hailstorm, the pitta fire is completely blown out. The digestive fire can't metabolize food, emotions, or thoughts. The whole mind-body is in a continuous state of alarm and feels undernourished and exhausted.

The causes for the initial vata imbalance are endless—mental or emotional stress, overwork, overstimulation, understimulation, wrong foods, irregular habits, insomnia—and need to be addressed for permanent, long-term results.

Also see Depression, Insomnia, and Menopause Symptoms.

AYURVEDA

AYURVEDIC SELF-CARE

Follow the Daily Lifestyle Regimen that will balance vata. Watch your diet. Eating too much, especially fatty foods or refined carbohydrates, can make you feel lethargic, as can inadequate vitamins and minerals, particularly not enough of the B-vitamins, iron, manganese, phosphorus, and potassium. Anemia (for example from poor diet or loss of too much blood during menstruation) may lead to fatigue and low energy. Make every effort to kick the caffeine habit. One of the first things people do to combat fatigue is to give themselves an artificial lift by reaching for the coffee, tea, colas, or other caffeinated beverages. These are not only health busters if you rely on them too regularly, but they actually set you up for a late-in-the-day letdown. If taken too late at night, they'll ruin your sleep, tempting you to perk up in the morning with another couple of cups and setting you up for a vicious cycle. Better to start the day with vata tea, meditation, and by giving yourself an abhyanga massage.

Get active. If your get-up-and-go "got up and went," you'll be amazed at the energizing powers of regular vigorous exercise. Lying around like a couch potato or desk potato doesn't conserve energy, as some people think—it actually makes you more tired and lethargic. It may seem difficult to bestir yourself if you've been in a low-energy slump for some time, but for many people, once they start, they have just as much trouble stopping as they did starting because they feel so much peppier. Yoga calms vata, and the Thunderbolt Pose is also particularly recommended.

Get busy. If understimulation could be a root cause of your lack of energy, the answer is to get involved and don't wait for your partner to go with you or share your activities. It's your responsibility to take care of your own needs for more stimulation, so get out there and mingle, or join, or take a class, or start politicking for better schools, or better government, or whatever.

THE A-Z GUIDE

HERBAL REMEDIES

- For exhaustion, take 1 teaspoon brahmi (gotu kola) with 1 cup warm milk as needed.

- For fatigue and weakness, combine 1 teaspoon jatamansi (Nardostachys jatamansi), 1 teaspoon ghee, and 1 teaspoon honey; take twice a day.

- The Ten-Day Ginger Treatment is one of the best ways to stimulate the digestive fire so that you can metabolize all your experiences and provide your mind-body with the nourishment it needs to feel energetic again.

FIVE-SENSE THERAPIES

- Taste: Emphasize tastes that are sweet, pungent, and salty.

- Smell: Use vata-calming aromas that are warm, sweet, and sour, such as cloves, orange, rose geranium, and basil.

- Sight: Red color therapy restores energy.

- Hearing: Listen to the late afternoon raga between the hours of four and seven P.M.

- Touch: Abhyanga, which calms vata and stimulates many marma points, is the best touch therapy for fatigue.

IMPORTANT PRECAUTIONS FOR FATIGUE

Chronic or overwhelming fatigue that doesn't respond to the self-care approaches suggested here may signal any number of underlying serious conditions, including anemia, hypoglycemia, diabetes, hypothyroidism, or chronic fatigue syndrome, that you should have evaluated professionally. However, your doctor may not be prepared to hunt down and treat the less threatening causes of vague symptoms such as fatigue. These include: exhaustion of your adrenal glands (for example, from too much stress); environmental or food allergies; sensitivities; a burned-out immune system; and problems with assimilating food. Immune dysfunctions may allow systemic infection such as yeast infection and the flourishing of common viruses, which often include fatigue as the initial overwhelming symptom.

FEVER

Fever is usually a symptom that a viral or bacterial infection has taken hold; these include colds, flu, earaches, diarrhea, cystitis, and common childhood diseases such as chicken pox, mumps, and measles. Although fever may be the only sign, or the major symptom, of an illness (especially during the early stage), the height of a person's temperature does not necessarily indicate the seriousness of the disease.

Fever, like all symptoms, has long been considered by Ayurveda and other natural medicines to be a positive sign that the body is defending itself from infection. Mild sweating is helpful to release ama, the buildup of toxins that get in the way of health and healing. Conventional medicine is finally realizing that fever has many beneficial functions. It speeds the metabolism so that more blood, oxygen, and nutrients are available and waste products are carried away more quickly. The extra heat slows down the invading organism and makes it more vulnerable to the germ-fighting components of the immune system. This powerful natural defense mechanism is usually not a cause for concern and in most cases it should be left alone to do its job during an acute illness.

Ayurveda says that fever is caused by a universal dosha imbalance, which destabilizes the temperature gauge in the body. Self-care helps keep you more comfortable and supports the healing efforts of the body. In certain circumstances a well-chosen Ayurvedic remedy offers a safe, effective

THE A-Z GUIDE

way to reduce a fever by helping it to be a more effective healing tool. Consider adding an Ayurvedic remedy if: the fever is very high for a prolonged period of time (over 102 degrees F for more than an hour, or reaches 104 degrees F); a child has had a febrile seizure in the past; or the person is becoming depleted from the fever or is very uncomfortable.

(Note: If a child has a febrile seizure, do not become unduly alarmed. Seizures usually last only 1 to 5 minutes and rarely last longer than 20 or 30 minutes or cause permanent harm. Seizures are the body's reaction to a fever, which in certain children causes the brain to send inappropriate signals to the muscles. The body may stiffen, the hands and feet may beat rhythmically, the eyes may roll back and the head jerk.)

If the fever accompanies other distinct conditions and symptoms, refer to those sections as well, such as Colds and Flu.

AYURVEDIC SELF-CARE

Protect yourself from drafts and make sure you don't become chilled. Learn how to take a temperature to confirm and evaluate the severity of a fever. Oral thermometers work best for most individuals; rectal thermometers or axillary thermometers (armpit) work best for young children. Rest and drinking plenty of fluids support the body's healing efforts and replace fluids lost through sweating. A poor appetite is to be expected, so do not force foods. Small, bland, easily digestible meals are best, and avoid milk.

HERBAL REMEDIES

- Drink hot tea made with fresh grated ginger, fennel, honey, and lemon every half hour. In addition you may take one of the following:

- Mix 1/2 teaspoon triphala with 1/4 cup aloe vera juice; drink three times a day.

AYURVEDA

- Mix 1/2 teaspoon each triphala and lemongrass with 1 cup hot water; drink as a tea three times a day.

- Mix 1/8 teaspoon black pepper and 1/2 teaspoon tulsi with 1 cup hot water; take three times a day.

FIVE-SENSE THERAPIES

- Taste: Favor foods, herbs, and spices that are sweet, bitter, and astringent. Kicharee, a healing meal, is recommended as the basic solid food during a fever; sprinkle it with the summer churna.

- Smell: Sweet, cool aromas such as sandalwood, rose, mint, cinnamon, and jasmine are appropriate.

- Sight: Blue and orange color therapy soothes a fever.

- Hearing: Listen to the sunset raga between the hours of seven and ten P.M., or the midday raga between one and four P.M.

- Touch: Apply cool ginger compresses to the feet, navel, and forehead.

IMPORTANT PRECAUTIONS FOR FEVER

NEVER give aspirin to a child who has fever that may be due to chicken pox, as aspirin increases the risk of a serious liver and brain disease known as Reye's syndrome. Medical care should be sought if: a baby under 6 months of age has a fever; an older baby has had a fever for more than 24 hours that hasn't responded to Ayurvedic home care or remedies; the fever is over 105 degrees F in a person of any age; a child has had a febrile seizure during a past or the current illness; there are signs of dehydration.

THE A-Z GUIDE

FIRST AID FOR INJURIES

No home is complete without a good first-aid manual. In addition to the standard recommended steps for common injuries, you may use the following Ayurvedic remedies. Be sure to consult a health care professional if the injury is serious 'or if it doesn't respond to first aid.

BITES

- For bites and stings from insects, snakes, or animals:

- Make a juice from 2 bundles fresh cilantro and 4 apples; drink 2 ounces of this every 2 hours.

- Make a paste of 1/4 teaspoon turmeric, 1 1/2 teaspoons water, and a little Neem oil; apply to the affected area.

BRUISES

- For painful black-and-blue marks:

- Apply Mahagenesh oil directly on the bruise.

BURNS

- For a first-degree burn, such as most sunburns, or second-degree burns that are not extensive:

- Mix 1/2 teaspoon turmeric powder with 1 teaspoon aloe vera gel and apply to the affected area continuously.

CUTS AND SCRAPES

- For minor cuts, scrapes, and all types of wounds (except deep puncture wounds):

- Mix 1/2 teaspoon turmeric powder with 1 teaspoon aloe vera gel and apply to the affected area until redness and swelling subside.

DENTAL TRAUMA

Ayurvedic remedies can ease pain and avoid problems after traumatic dental procedures such as root canal or tooth extraction, or pain and inflammation surrounding the eruption of wisdom teeth. The most common Ayurvedic remedies for dental trauma are the following:

- Apply clove oil to the gums.

- Gargle with 1/4 teaspoon triphala mixed with 1/2 cup warm water.

- Gargle with warm sesame oil.

- Suck on a whole clove.

HEAT EXHAUSTION

Signs of overheating, heat exhaustion, or heat stress are dizziness, fainting, or giddiness; excessive sweating; cold, moist, pale skin; thirst; extreme weakness or fatigue; headache; nausea and vomiting; muscle cramps; and a rapid, weak pulse. Choose one of the following Ayurvedic treatments for heat exhaustion:

- Drink 1 cup coconut milk or grape juice.

- Add 3 dates to 1 cup water and boil; blend and drink.

THE A-Z GUIDE

- Drink fresh cilantro juice every 6 hours; add 1/2 teaspoon manjishta (Rubio cordifolium).

MUSCLE INJURY

When we injure a muscle through overwork or overstretching, the tiny fibers that make up the "meat" of the muscle are torn. The following Ayurvedic remedy helps speed healing and ease pain and stiffness:

- Put 1 tablespoon of mustard oil on a cloth compress you have dipped in hot water and wrung out, and fold the cloth so the oil does not come into direct contact with the skin. Apply for 20 minutes, or until the pain starts to subside.

SHOCK

Shock is common after an injury or allergic reaction. The symptoms are: pale or "ashen" skin; perspiration; dilated (wide-open) pupils; the person also appears to be lethargic, acts "shocky," or loses consciousness, takes shallow or irregular breaths, and has a weak pulse or heart rate. Shock is a medical emergency and requires immediate professional care; in the meantime Ayurveda can help minimize and reverse the symptoms:

- Inhale freshly sliced onion or calamus root powder

STRAINS AND SPRAINS

Under conditions of overuse or strong force, ligaments and tendons can be overstretched, resulting in a strain; or they may be partially torn, resulting in a sprain. (Complete tears are rare.) These connective-tissue injuries generally take four to six weeks to heal, and home care and Ayurveda can ease the process. The most common Ayurvedic remedies for strains and sprains are to:

- Apply a mustard oil or castor oil compress to the injury.

- Massage Mahanarayan on the lower back; this medicated oil consisting of approximately ten herbs in a sesame oil base, is commonly used to treat musculoskeletal problems.

FLATULENCE (GAS)

Flatulence is gas that has formed in the stomach and bowels by swallowed air, poor diet, or eating a food or combination of foods that are not easily digested. As a result the gas is eventually expelled through the anus, which may relieve any stomach discomfort that accompanies the flatulence.

In Ayurveda gas is considered to be a vata disorder in which there is a vata imbalance in the gastrointestinal area. If your body doesn't have strong enough enzymes, it cannot break down food. This disrupts the normal peristalsis (muscle movement) in the intestines, causing gas to form. If you have gas frequently it is a sure sign that you aren't getting all you could from your food.

Also see Indigestion.

AYURVEDIC SELF-CARE

If you are bothered by intestinal gas, incorporate the following specific remedies into your Daily Lifestyle Regimen. Yoga may also be helpful, particularly Rocking and Rolling and Leg Lock Pose.

HERBAL REMEDIES

- Begin by taking 1/2 teaspoon triphala with 1/2 cup warm water; drink at bedtime. In addition choose one or both of the following:

THE A-Z GUIDE

- Mix together equal parts ashwagandha, shatavari (Asparagus racemosus), and shankhapushpi (Crotalaria verrucosa); take 1/2 teaspoon of this mixture with 1/2 cup

- Warm water in the early evening.

- Mix 1/2 teaspoon each fennel and cumin with 1 cup hot water; drink as a tea in the early morning.

- For relief of acute gas episodes, try one of the following remedies:

- Drink 1/2 teaspoon cumin mixed in 1 cup hot water.

- Drink 1 pinch hingu mixed with 1 teaspoon ghee and follow with warm water.

FIVE-SENSE THERAPIES

- Taste: Incorporate more sweet, sour, and salty tastes into your diet. Using the winter churna every day is an easy way to do this.

- Smell: Use sweet, warm aromas as your aromatherapy, such as basil, orange, rose geranium, and cloves.

- Sight: Yellow-green color therapy is particularly effective in minimizing flatulence.

- Hearing: Listen to the late-afternoon raga between four and seven P.M.

- Touch: Apply sesame oil to your lower abdomen and massage in a clockwise direction three times a day. Apply Brahmi oil to the marma point known as Kukundara.

AYURVEDA

IMPORTANT PRECAUTIONS FOR FLATULENCE

If Ayurvedic remedies do not provide relief of acute gas within 1 day, or of chronic gas within 2 weeks, consult a health care professional.

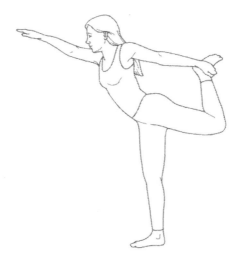

Lord Shiva's Pose: Stand straight and tall. Shift your weight to your right foot and bend your left leg back until you can grab your left foot or ankle with your left hand. Raise your right arm and reach up and out; tip your upper body slightly forward as you extend your left foot out. Hold the pose as long as possible, breathing deeply and evenly and gazing at a point in front of you for balance. Slowly release and repeat with the other leg.

FOOD CRAVINGS

Some people crave rich chocolate, some gotta have sour crunchy pickles even when they're not pregnant. Others devour fresh yeasty bread or are addicted to the crisp saltiness of potato chips. Whatever the craving, Ayurveda considers this condition to be .a mistake of the intellect. According to this thinking, eating certain foods habitually will produce toxins that clog and imbalance your system rather than nourish your body

THE A-Z GUIDE

and create health. Some Western allergists believe that food addiction is the first sign of a food allergy. The biochemical change caused by ingesting the food gives you a sense of well-being, and when this wears off, you need the food again.

AYURVEDIC SELF-CARE

Follow the appropriate Daily Lifestyle Regimen for balancing your doshas. The yoga posture called Lord Shiva's Pose, is particularly useful for relieving this condition. The most effective way to begin to break the cycle of craving is to introduce all six tastes with churna and do a weekly fast. After following this program for three months, your brain chemistry will re-regulate itself, freeing you from your cravings.

- Six-Taste Therapy: Simply get the churna appropriate for your dosha and sprinkle some on your food at every meal. The six tastes supply the variety that humans crave and seek to fulfill (in a perverted way) through cravings and that our culture seeks to fulfill through 10 different kinds of cornflakes, 100 flavored iced teas, 27 different salad dressings, and 132 kinds of fat-free cookies.

- In addition one day a week go on the Juice-and-Soup Fast, drinking only fruit and vegetable juices and soup.

HERBAL REMEDIES

- You may take 1/2 teaspoon triphala with 1/2 cup warm water at bedtime daily.

- Combine 5 parts shatavari (Asparagus racemosus), 2 parts tikta, 2 parts kama, and 3 parts guduchi (Tinospora cordifolia); take 1/4 teaspoon twice daily following lunch and dinner.

AYURVEDA

FIVE-SENSE THERAPIES

- Taste: Make sure you are getting all six tastes by using the six-taste therapy.

- Smell: Sweet, cool aromas such as jasmine, sandalwood, and mint help reduce cravings.

- Sight: Blue-green color therapy is said to be effective.

- Hearing: Listen to the sunset raga between the hours of seven and ten P.M.

- Touch: Apply one drop of warm sesame oil to the marma point known as Brahma Randhra, on the top of the skull, 3 finger widths in front of the point of the crown; apply finger pressure for 60 seconds. Repeat three to four times a day.

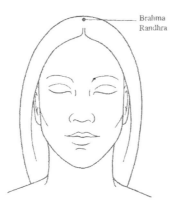

The manna point for food cravings: Brahma Randhra.

THE A-Z GUIDE

IMPORTANT PRECAUTIONS FOR FOOD CRAVINGS

If you still experience cravings after Ayurvedic self-care, consult a physician; food cravings may be due to food allergy or nutritional deficiency. You should also seek medical care if you overeat and then force yourself to vomit.

FUNGUS INFECTION/CANDIDA

Modern names for common afflictions such as candida (or herpes, or eczema and others) were not precisely named in the ancient Sanskrit Ayurvedic texts. However, there were treatises on different "bugs"— infectious agents such as funguses that invade the system and cause a general weakness, skin disorders, and nervous system imbalances, much like the current symptoms attributed to Candida albicans, a yeast-like fungus. Like most infectious agents, Candida is usually harmless and is normally found in the mouth, digestive tract, vagina, and on the skin of healthy people. It is only when your resistance is low that it can overgrow and cause problems such as diaper rash, thrush, and vaginitis.

Also see Vaginitis.

AYURVEDIC SELF-CARE

As is the case with all systemic infections, the Ayurvedic method of restoring balance to the mind-body is multifaceted. It consists of purifying the system, applying local treatment if necessary, and restrengthening your defenses. Follow the program presented below for at least 6 months and up to one year; yeast is cantankerous, tenacious, and hard to evict.

Step 1. Bioenergetic Water Treatment. Boil pure water for 10 minutes, let cool, and drink 1 to 2 ounces every half hour or hour. Do this for three days to loosen the accumulated ama.

AYURVEDA

Step 2. Take 1/2 teaspoon triphala and 1/4 teaspoon trikatu with vata tea. Do this for the next three days to increase agni (digestive fire) and cleanse the bowels.

Step 3. Do the Juice-and-Soup Fast for 2 days to further cleanse your system.

Step 4. Restrengthen the system with a mixture of 1/4 teaspoon each turmeric (an antifungal) and ghee, taken once a day; for 3 days also take 1/2 teaspoon mahasudar Shan mixed with V2 cup warm water. Do this for 1 week, then stop for 1 week, then begin again with step 1.

HERBAL REMEDIES

- In addition to the above program, use one of the following:

- For skin infection: Apply turmeric powder to the affected area.

- For toenail or fingernail fungus: Mix together 1/2 teaspoon each aloe vera gel and turmeric powder; apply this paste to the entire nail area.

- For fungal infection of the ear. Use garlic oil. Turn your head to the side and pour 1/4 teaspoon of the oil into the affected ear; keep head in place for 5 minutes, then place a small piece of cotton in the ear to hold the oil in place for 10 minutes. Do this once a day for 2 weeks.

FIVE-SENSE THERAPIES

- Taste: Make sure you have bitter and astringent tastes in your diet; bitter melon is an excellent source, available where Chinese groceries are sold.

- Smell: Use bitter, warm, and sweet aromas.

THE A-Z GUIDE

- Sight: Orange color therapy will support the immune system.

- Hearing: Listen to the late-afternoon and sunset ragas during the appropriate hours.

- Touch: Massage oregano oil into the fungal infection.

IMPORTANT PRECAUTIONS FOR
FUNGUS INFECTION/CANDIDA

If symptoms persist, seek medical care.

GRIEF AND SADNESS

Grief and sadness are part of everyone's life because at some point we all lose someone or something we care about. It could be the death of a loved one or a pet; the loss of a job and thus our income and identity; the end of a relationship and thus the loss of a spouse, child, lover, or friend; we may be the victim of a violent crime, such as a rape or mugging; we may need to move away from our home and experience the grief called homesickness.

Unexpressed grief and sadness affect the vata dosha, which vibrates with grief. According to Ayurveda, if these feelings remain unresolved, they accumulate in the lower gut, the neck, the circulatory system, and the mind. Not surprisingly kapha types tend to cope with grief the best, because their groundedness equips them to absorb such emotional shocks.

Ayurveda has several remedies that support our own healing efforts during times of such acute crisis. These remedies are able to soothe us when our feelings are still new and thus the most raw and painful. The

AYURVEDA

expression of these natural feelings helps heal the injury of the loss and releases us to face the future with better balance.

AYURVEDIC SELF-CARE

We all have different ways and different timetables for recovering from important losses. Some of us bounce back right away; others need more time to heal. There is no "right" way, but the following suggestions have helped many people weather the emotional storm:

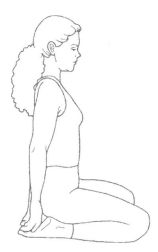

Intoxicating Bliss Pose: Sit on your feet, knees apart. Place your hands on your heels, palms facing downward on the soles of your feet. Inhale and exhale deeply and slowly, concentrating on the breath, and stay in this position for as long as is comfortable.

As with all symptoms, suppressing grief and sadness is not healthy in the long run. Generally it is better to acknowledge your loss and talk about it to another person or persons in a safe, supportive environment.

Remember, emotions help you heal, so don't "beat yourself up" for feeling the way you do. Take the time to pray, meditate, contemplate, and honor your loss.

THE A-Z GUIDE

The more important and deeper the feeling of grief, the more likely that unhealed losses in the past are being stirred up. But even this can be helpful because

it brings up issues that are still bothering you and should be dealt with in order to restore balance.

Listen to your own individual needs: Do you feel better when you are left alone or when you are in the company of others? Might you find comfort in talking to people who share similar experiences and feelings? If so, seek out a support group or peer counselor who understands what you are going through. Often short-term counseling is all a person needs to get through a difficult period.

Practicing yoga is recommended to restore balance and to help you feel and express emotions you might be having trouble letting out. The Intoxicating Bliss Pose, is particularly recommended during times of sadness and grief.

HERBAL REMEDIES

- Combine 1/4 teaspoon arjuna (Terminalia arjuna) and 1/2 teaspoon each saraswati and triphala; take 1/2 teaspoon of this mixture in vata tea.

FIVE-SENSE THERAPIES

- Taste: Emphasize sweet, sour, and salty tastes at this time. A simple way to do this is to flavor your food with winter churna every day.

- Smell: Sweet, warm aromas such as rose, basil, orange, jasmine, and clary sage are soothing.

- Sight: Violet, blue, and green are recommended for color therapy.

- Hearing: Listen to the sunrise and sunset ragas during the appropriate times of day.

- Touch: Daily sesame oil massage (abhyanga) is very important all the time, but can be extremely helpful during these periods in your life.

IMPORTANT PRECAUTIONS FOR GRIEF AND SADNESS

Seek medical care if crisis symptoms last for more than a week, or if you show signs of depression (see Depression).

HAY FEVER

The nose, throat, and eyes are often targets for airborne allergens; as a result of exposure, you sneeze (sometimes intensely and uncontrollably), your nose and eyes run and are unbearably itchy, or your nose may be stuffy; sometimes even the roof of your mouth or your ears itch too.

In many people the problem stems from high levels of pollen—tiny grains released by plants, trees, and grasses—and so is confined to certain times of the year. Such "hay fever" usually occurs in the late summer or fall and spring; but this depends on the geographical location and climate patterns. Dust, molds, and animal dander (from pets or feather bedding) are also frequent upper respiratory allergens.

From the Ayurvedic perspective allergies arise when agents that have made their way into the nasal passages irritate the brain chemistry. This in turn leads to a deranged immune response. If you are very sensitive, the antibody-antigen complex becomes overstimulated and clogs your system. Since hay fever is a chronic, deep-seated condition, the self-care suggestions given below will provide only temporary relief; a true cure requires a skilled professional knowledgeable in Ayurveda. You may want to consider going to a clinic that specializes in pancha karma, or purification techniques.

THE A-Z GUIDE

AYURVEDIC SELF-CARE

Following the appropriate Daily Lifestyle Routine will help balance your doshas and normalize your immune system. When practicing yoga, add the Lion Pose, which may help clear air passages. The following steps may also help lessen or avoid symptoms:

Try to avoid the things that trigger hay fever, such as pollen, animal dander, or dust. Avoid heavily planted areas during hay fever season and keep your home as dust-free as possible. Use an air cleaner in bedrooms. Take up carpets and use synthetic fiber pillows and blankets.

Rinse your face (nose, eyes) with cool water and wash hands when you get home; wash hair frequently. These measures remove pollen and other allergens that cling to your body.

If breathing is difficult because of swollen nasal passages, inhale water vapor from a humidifier to open them up.

If eyes are very irritated, rinse them periodically with sterile saline solution (salt water available at drugstores) to dislodge pollen and soothe inflamed membranes.

HERBAL REMEDIES

- These remedies help protect and strengthen the nasal passages and increase the digestive fire so that you can better shrug off the assailants.

- Combine 2 drops each of ghee and Brahmi oil and sniff three times a day.

- Or you may do nasaya (nasal-passage lubrication) with sesame oil three to five times a day.

AYURVEDA

- Combine 1/4 teaspoon sitopladi and 1/8 teaspoon trikatu; take with 1/2 cup warm water three times a day if symptoms are severe.

- Drink a tea made from 1/4 teaspoon fresh grated ginger and honey and lemon to taste twice a day.

FIVE-SENSE THERAPIES

- Taste: Be sure to include pungent, bitter, and astringent tastes in your diet; a convenient way to do this is with spring chuma.

- Smell: Warm, spicy aromas are useful in dispelling hay fever symptoms.

- Sight Red and orange color therapy is recommended.

- Hearing: Listen to the sunset raga between the hours of seven and ten P.M.

- Touch: Add 1 drop clove oil to 3 teaspoons sesame oil; apply a drop of this mixture and finger pressure to the marina points.

IMPORTANT PRECAUTIONS FOR HAY FEVER

If symptoms persist or are severe, consult a health practitioner.

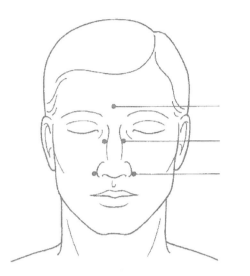

Anja

Ganda

Nasa

The manna points for hay fever: Ajna, Ganda, and Nasa.

HOARSENESS

Hoarseness is a symptom of laryngitis, an inflammation of the mucous membrane lining the voice box (larynx) that causes a swelling of the vocal cords. This acute condition may arise during an upper respiratory infection such as a cold or from overuse of the voice.

In Ayurveda the throat is thought to be the bridge between the heart and the mind. Your throat muscles express emotions by producing sound; these emotional events are recorded in the muscle tissue. Hoarseness is therefore considered to be a vata imbalance that over taxes the laryngeal muscles, glands, and organs of the throat.

Chronic laryngitis is usually due to chronic overuse or incorrect use of the voice or to smoking. It may also be a sign of serious disease.

AYURVEDA

Therefore chronic laryngitis requires professional evaluation and advice about learning to use vocal cords correctly, or less vocalizing, stopping smoking, or medical treatment.

If laryngitis accompanies other cold symptoms such as a cough or sore throat, refer to those sections in the book for additional information about self-care and Ayurvedic remedies.

AYURVEDIC SELF-CARE

Follow the Daily Lifestyle Regimen to balance your dosha, especially if you have chronic hoarseness. Alternate-nostril breathing helps calm vata, as does yoga, the Thunderbolt Pose in particular. To soothe the inflamed larynx and encourage healing, inhale steam from a vaporizer, humidifier, or bowl of heated water. Rest the voice as much as possible and gargle with 1/4 teaspoon sesame oil mixed with 1 cup warm water. Drinking liquids may help ease pain; pittas usually prefer cold while vatas and kaphas prefer warm beverages.

HERBAL REMEDIES

Mix 1/2 teaspoon each cinnamon and licorice with 1 teaspoon honey; place a small amount in your mouth and let dissolve slowly.

FIVE SENSE THERAPIES

- Taste: Emphasize sweet, sour, and salty tastes; the winter churna provides these tastes.

- Smell: Inhale sweet, warm aromas such as cloves, orange, and basil.

- Sight: Yellow-green is the color therapy to use.

- Hearing: Listen to the midday or late-afternoon raga during the appropriate hours.

THE A-Z GUIDE

- Touch: Apply one drop of warm sesame oil and finger pressure to the marma points shown below.

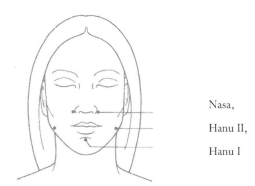

Nasa,

Hanu II,

Hanu I

The marma points for hoarseness: Nasa, Hanu II, and Hanu I.

IMPORTANT PRECAUTIONS FOR HOARSENESS

Seek medical care if: swallowing is very painful; there is excessive dribbling of saliva or breathing problems in a young child; the laryngitis lasts more than 7 days.

HYPERACTIVITY AND ATTENTION DEFICIT DISORDER (ADD)

This is a condition that affects children, teenagers, and sometimes adults. Symptoms may be mild or severe and include blocked vision, language, memory, and motor skills; short attention span; impulsiveness; emotional instability; and sometimes physical over-activity. It is ten times more common among boys than it is among girls. The standard Western therapy is the drug Ritalin, and 96 percent of the Ritalin used in the world is prescribed in the United States.

This is a sobering statistic, and considering this, we must ask, why are American children so much more afflicted than children in other parts of the world? Conventional medicine is at a loss to explain the phenomenon; it guesses that this nervous system condition is due to genetic factors, a chemical imbalance, or injury or disease at or after birth.

Ayurveda asks, is it something in our culture and environment? Is it perhaps the preponderance of junky, processed sweet and salty food we eat; the unceasing inundation of stimulation via TV, video, computers, and electronic games; the lack of exposure to nature, physical exercise, and other healthy outlets for childhood exuberance, enthusiasm, and curiosity?

ADD has all the signs of a vata imbalance. It should come as no surprise that well-regarded, well-traveled Ayurveda practitioners have noticed that in the United States, patients of all ages always have some level of vata imbalance; even in other highly technical societies such as Canada and France, there is far less vata imbalance. Not only have they not fallen into the trap of overstimulation but their cultural traditions follow the natural rhythms of the day, so they practice healthier patterns of activity and rest. In France it is still common to take two-hour lunch breaks rather than gobbling a sandwich and chips at one's desk. Kids don't rush frantically from activity to activity, and have more quiet time with the family. Rather than drugging our children, we must therefore work at calming the nervous system, nourishing the nerve tissue, and feeding the brain.

AYURVEDIC SELF-CARE

Reconsider the level and quality of stimulation in your family's life. Help your child follow the Daily Lifestyle Regimen that will balance his or her doshas, practice yoga together (there are books on yoga for children, who enjoy the animal names of many of the poses), and incorporate the following specific remedies.

THE A-Z GUIDE

HERBAL REMEDIES

- Start with 1/2 teaspoon triphala with 1/2 cup warm water each night before bedtime, then add one of the following:

- Mix together 4 parts ashwaghanda (Withania somnifera), 2 parts shatavari (Asparagus racemosus), and 1 part jatamansi (Nordostachys jatamansi). Take the following amount of this combination, with 1/2 cup warm milk, depending on your age: Child, 2 pinches; teenager, 1/8 teaspoon; adult, 1/4 to 1/2 teaspoon. Take once a day, and if the results are not adequate, take twice a day.

FIVE-SENSE THERAPIES

- Taste: Use the winter churna sprinkled on food, as well as other whole foods with sweet, salty, and sour tastes.

- Smell: Use aromatherapy that is sweet and warm, such as rose, clary sage, basil, and orange.

- Sight: Green and yellow color therapy is beneficial, especially the green found in nature.

- Hearing: Music therapy helps children calm down and focus, so let them listen to the sunrise, midmorning, and midday ragas during the appropriate times of day. Why not ask the teacher to play it in the classroom?

- Touch: The most important step to take is to massage your child with warm sesame oil every day.

IMPORTANT PRECAUTIONS FOR HYPERACTIVITY

If symptoms persist despite Ayurvedic treatment, have your child examined by an allergist. Allergies have been linked with many of the

AYURVEDA

symptoms of hyperactivity, and allergies are treatable if properly diagnosed, such as with NAET (Namudripad Allergy Elimination Technique).

HYPERTENSION

Hypertension is a persistently elevated level of blood pressure in your main arteries. Blood pressure is considered to be normal if it is between 140/85 and 120/70. High blood pressure has no noticeable symptoms and it often goes undetected; yet it can have very severe complications including heart attack and stroke.

Hypertension is often a symptom of another disease. It is a classic pitta disorder, but each of the three doshas has its own unique way of expressing hypertension. In a vata imbalance, hypertension is erratic and the blood pressure goes up and down and is related to the events and worries in your life. Pittas with high blood pressure have red faces, red eyes, are irritable, have a general burning sensation, and heartburn is common. In kapha types, the blood pressure stays high; you retain water, feel lethargic, and may have swollen joints.

High blood pressure requires prompt medical attention. The conventional wisdom is to reduce salt and excess fat in your diet and engage in regular aerobic exercise. In Ayurveda, managing high blood pressure requires that you treat the underlying imbalance through lifestyle and specific remedies.

AYURVEDIC SELF-CARE

Following the Daily Lifestyle Regimen for balancing your doshas over the long term will help normalize blood pressure. Meditation has been shown to lower blood pressure in people considered to be borderline hypertensives. This is very significant because half of the people who die of hypertension-related deaths are in the borderline category. Also important are alternate-nostril breathing, yoga Sun Salutations, and the yoga pose known as the Intoxicating Bliss Pose. You may also add the following specific remedies.

HERBAL REMEDIES

- For persistent hypertension: Combine 5 parts punarnava (Boerrhavia diffusa), 3 parts saraswati, 2 parts jatamansi (Nordostachys jatamans), and 2 parts brahmi (gotu kola); take 3/4 teaspoon of this mixture mixed with 1/2 cup warm water twice a day.

- For a tendency to hypertension: Mix 1/2 teaspoon arjuna (Terminalia arjuna) with 1/4 teaspoon triphala; add 1 teaspoon honey (for kaphas) or ghee (for pittas) or half milk and ghee (for vatas). Take this as daily tonic in the morning for 2 weeks of every month.

FIVE-SENSE THERAPIES

- Taste: Emphasize sweet, bitter, and astringent tastes in your diet; the summer churna is a handy way to accomplish this.

- Smell: Use aromatherapy with essential oils that smell sweet and cool, such as jasmine, mint, and sandalwood.

- Sight: Blue or indigo color therapy helps normalize blood pressure.

- Hearing: Listen to the midmorning raga between the hours of ten A.M. and one P.M.

- Touch: Daily sesame oil massage helps lower blood pressure.

IMPORTANT PRECAUTIONS FOR HYPERTENSION

If hypertension is persistent, you must be under medical care.

AYURVEDA

HYPOGLYCEMIA

Hypoglycemia occurs when you have too little sugar in your blood. As a result you feel weak, headachy, hungry, and anxious; you may have problems with your vision, lose your muscle coordination, and have personality changes. The usual explanation is that the pancreas is releasing too much insulin, which lowers the sugar in the blood, or you that are eating too little food.

In Ayurveda low blood sugar is considered to be one of many imbalances of the digestive system. It is a classic piṭṭa disorder because the agni, or digestive fire, isn't strong enough. Without a strong digestion or a properly regulated metabolism, your small intestine can't work properly.

AYURVEDIC SELF-CARE

Ayurveda seeks to restore digestive health to normalize blood sugar levels. Be sure to follow the Daily Lifestyle Regimen to balance your doshas and improve the strength of your agni. Beyond these basic measures, the first specific step you can take is to eat fresh grated ginger, which you may add to warm water to make a tea, before the midday meal to enhance your digestion. Then you may also add the following remedies.

HERBAL REMEDIES

- Do the Ten-Day Ginger Treatment at the beginning of every month.

- Twice a week, drink 1 cup juice made with cilantro, dandelion greens, cumin, and apples to taste.

FIVE-SENSE THERAPIES

- Taste: Favor sweet, bitter, pungent tastes in your food, herbs, and spices. Use the summer churna daily.

- Smell: Sweet, cool aromas are helpful, such as sandalwood, rose, mint, cinnamon, and jasmine.

- Sight: Choose blue and indigo for your color therapy.

- Hearing: Listen to the ragas composed for the hours from ten A.M. to one P.M.

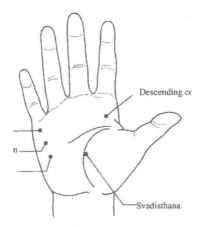

The manna points for hypoglycemia: Descending colon, Liver, Transverse colon, Ascending colon, and Svadisthana.

- Touch: Apply one drop of warm sesame oil and clockwise finger pressure to the marma points, three times a day. This stimulates the digestive organs.

IMPORTANT PRECAUTIONS FOR HYPOGLYCEMIA

Hypoglycemia, if left untreated, may lead to delirium, coma, and death. If you have the symptoms of low blood sugar, be sure to see a health care professional for an accurate diagnosis and treatment.

AYURVEDA

INDIGESTION

Almost everyone feels some digestive system discomfort at one time or another. Bouts of acute indigestion may result from eating too much or too fast, or eating rich foods, or emphasizing the wrong foods for your dosha or time of year. Emotional stress may initiate or worsen digestive problems. The Western view of indigestion—gas, pain, bloating—is treated with antacids designed to reduce the acidity in your stomach. Then it's on to the next meal to begin the eat-pain-medication cycle all over again.

Ayurveda takes a larger view. Indigestion is considered to be an imbalance of all three doshas. It is also the starting point for many other complicated disorders. To understand indigestion, you have to understand digestion. Your body secretes agni, the innate digestive energy or digestive juices that must be healthy, strong, and full of live metabolic enzymes in order to break down the food, thoughts, feelings, and events of the day so that no ama is left to clog the passageways.

However, if these juices are weak, lacking in volume (about eight quarts a day are secreted), concentration, or have an acid imbalance, your body cannot break down the needed nutrients. As a result it feels undernourished; it becomes weak, and a vicious cycle develops wherein a weak body produces weak digestive juices, which makes the body weaker, and so on. If your fire is low and tissues are not nourished, the ama starts accumulating. Undigested food, emotions, feelings, and thoughts allow bacteria to flourish and poison your system. If you have old ama that has been collecting for a long time, it leads to imbalances in assimilation, liver congestion, heart and emotional issues, and problems with your skin and eyes. Ayurveda offers relief for both chronic and acute indigestion. The most important step is to keep a good strong fire in the belly. You do this by eating foods rich in live enzymes, such as sprouts, greens, and fresh ginger.

The six tastes are the next important consideration in digestion. The mind-body requires all six tastes to turn on all the parts of the brain

THE A-Z GUIDE

every day. Through churna you can easily incorporate taste therapy into your life and achieve the simultaneous stimulation your brain requires for total nourishment. General recommendations for indigestion follow; for remedies for specific symptoms and related conditions, also see Abdominal Bloating, Abdominal Pain, Acid Stomach, Constipation, Diarrhea, Flatulence, Intestinal Pain, Motion Sickness, Nausea, and Ulcer, Stomach.

AYURVEDIC SELF-CARE

As you follow the Daily Lifestyle Regimen to balance your doshas, your digestive problems should even out. Make a special effort to eat regular meals, following the dietary guidelines for the three doshas. Avoid overeating, especially close to bedtime. Eating more slowly and being careful not to swallow air (don't talk while you eat, and don't argue!) will help most 'digestive problems such as indigestion and gas. So will eating small meals, perhaps six times a day, and eating slowly and chewing thoroughly.

Tension, anxiety, and other stress can cause situational intestinal cramps, gas, and diarrhea; chronic stress can also cause chronic diarrhea, stomach pains, and heartburn. So try to find ways to relax more often and manage the stress in your life. Stress and emotional upheaval can cause digestive upset during and between meals, so try to eat when you are relaxed. Meditation, yoga, and breathing exercises are also relaxing and help support agni. Massaging your whole lower and upper abdomen with Brahmi oil is a general digestive aid; lie down on your back and use twenty to thirty circular strokes daily until the indigestion subsides.

Remember, smoking tends to worsen heartburn and indigestion and in some people all they need to do to remedy digestive problems is to quit smoking.

Although strenuous exercise may not be appealing during times of digestive distress, regular strenuous exercise improves circulation, strengthens muscles, and is a potent antidote to stress— all of which are a boon to healthy digestion. Exercise, even walking, stimulates proper bowel function. A moderately paced walk among pleasant surroundings helps digestion and is particularly helpful in passing painful intestinal gas.

Other steps to take include the following:

- Avoid drinking icy-cold beverages during meals. Drink only small amounts of warm or room-temperature water with meals.

- Pay attention to the food combinations.

- Do not watch TV, read newspapers, or have intense conversations during dinner. Do not eat when driving.

- Eat all six tastes at least once every day, using the churna appropriate for your dosha.

- Eat fresh grated ginger with a pinch of salt before eating if you are having troublesome digestion.

- Eat mostly cooked foods.

- Eat heavy foods such as sweets early in the meal, when digestive juices are strongest, rather than later, when they are weaker.

HERBAL REMEDIES

- Add 2 pinches black pepper and 1 pinch hingu to 1 teaspoon ghee; take as needed.

- Combine 1 teaspoon shatavari (Asparagus racemosus) and 1/4 teaspoon each of kama and shankha bhasma; take 1/2 teaspoon of this mixture in 1/2 cup warm water three times daily, after meals.

THE A-Z GUIDE

- For chronic indigestion, take one of the following combinations with 1 cup warm water during a meal:

- 1 pinch ajwan (celery seed), 1 pinch hingu, 1/3 teaspoon cumin, 1/3 teaspoon fennel, and 1/2 teaspoon trikatu

- 1/3 teaspoon each cumin, coriander, and fennel

- 1/3 teaspoon each ginger, black pepper, pippali (long pepper), and cinnamon

- 1/4 teaspoon each shilajit, chitrak (Plumbago zeylonica), trikatu, punnarnava (Boerrhavia diffusa), guggul (Commiphora mukul), at lunch and dinner.

IMPORTANT PRECAUTIONS FOR INDIGESTION

Vague, chronic, or recurring abdominal pains in women may be due to pelvic infection or abnormal pregnancy. Chronic abdominal pain, especially if accompanied by other symptoms, should be evaluated by a professional. Indigestion is frequently confused with heart attack and can occur either during or after a large or spicy meal. So watch carefully the course of an attack of indigestion, especially if shortness of breath, sweating, or pain in the chest or arms is present. Better to have it checked out in an emergency room than to deny yourself measures that can save your life.

Frequent indigestion should always be mentioned to your health care professional since there are many digestive diseases that cause what we call indigestion: appendicitis, intestinal obstruction, and diseases of the gallbladder, pancreas, and intestines. Heartburn can be caused by ulcers, so if you have constant pain, particularly when your stomach is empty, ulcer disease should be ruled out.

AYURVEDA

INSOMNIA

Insomnia can become a chronic and vicious cycle. The less sleep you get, the less well you are able to deal with stress and the more difficult it is to fall or stay asleep. Chronic insomnia may also result from chronic anxiety, fear, tension, depression, and other psychological problems, drug abuse and dependence (including sleeping pills), or other chronic illness that causes nighttime symptoms of pain and distress.

In natural-medicine systems such as Ayurveda, sleep is one of the important components a person needs to restore and maintain physical and mental health. New studies show that chronic sleep deprivation, which may be due to insomnia, affects the immune system and our ability to stay alert and concentrate. Inadequate sleep may be responsible for poor productivity, irritability, and a large portion of accidents on the road, on the job, and at work.

If you are questioning the adequacy of your sleep, ask yourself, do I need an alarm clock to wake up every morning? If so, you are not getting adequate sleep. Do you wake up refreshed and energetic? If you are, then you needn't worry about getting enough sleep. Your "insomnia" means you are trying to fall asleep too early, or get up later than your body needs you to.

However, if you do suffer from occasional insomnia, or sleep fitfully and wake up tired, Ayurvedic self-care measures and remedies can help you restore a normal sleep schedule and awaken refreshed rather than exhausted. Instead of "knocking you out," as habit-forming conventional medicines tend to do, Ayurvedic practices and remedies encourage the body to drift into a natural, restful sleep.

Insomnia is a classic sign of a vata imbalance and a nervous system disorder. So many undigested life experiences can cause insomnia— career projects, family relationships, financial ventures, emotional upsets . . . the list goes on ad infinitum. The key is to treat the nervous system, which is on overdrive from too much stimulation.

THE A-Z GUIDE

AYURVEDIC SELF-CARE

Adopting a vata-stabilizing or pitta-stabilizing Daily Lifestyle Regimen will rebalance your doshas and go a long way toward restoring a healthy sleep pattern. In addition:

- The most important thing you can do to treat insomnia is to get to bed by ten P.M., every night, even on weekends. You need to establish a regular sleep pattern in order to be in sync with the chronobiology of your body cycles. Humans are preprogrammed to sleep soon after sunset and rise soon after sunrise. So if you ignore this, you are swimming against the tide of your biology, which is bound to create disturbed sleep.

- Avoid drinking alcoholic beverages in the evening. Although they may help you fall asleep initially, a few drinks before bedtime will actually awaken you in the middle of the night.

- Avoid caffeine (in coffee, black tea, sodas, chocolate, and some allopathic drugs) for several hours before bedtime. Some people are so sensitive to caffeine that even an afternoon cup of coffee keeps them up at night. Smoking also disturbs sleep.

- Create a bedtime ritual that cues your body for sleep and disengages the mind from daytime problems and thoughts. Relax by reading, taking a hot bath, or listening to music, particularly ragas. Yoga is also a good way to release the tensions of the day before bed, particularly the Cobra. Alternate-nostril breathing also calms the mind-body. Some people relax with friends; others find even lively conversation too stimulating. Watching TV may be relaxing but can also be stimulating, especially for children.

- Keep the bedroom for two things—sleep and sex. Using the bedroom for working overtime or paying bills signals the mind for activity, not relaxation. Some people find sex to be a pleasurable way to relax for sleep (although it could become habit-forming!).

- Diet can have a profound effect on your ability to sleep. Eat a light supper, not later than eight P.M. Eating dairy products, beets, carrots, and squash is very helpful for inducing sleep.

- Establish a regular exercise routine, but avoid exercise at night because it is stimulating.

- Some people find writing down the thoughts that are keeping them awake allows them to put the thoughts out of their minds long enough to fall asleep.

- Try using a relaxation technique such as meditation, which you can use both during the day and at night before retiring.

- Wear earplugs if your bedroom is noisy. Use a sleep mask and cover windows with heavy blinds or drapes if too much light comes through. Make sure the room temperature is comfortable and that there is adequate air circulation.

- Some people find daytime naps help; others find they make it more difficult to sleep at night, so experiment to see to which group you belong.

THE A-Z GUIDE

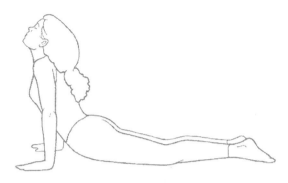

The Cobra: Lie flat on your stomach, elbows bent near your waist and palms of the hands at shoulder level on the floor. Inhale as you press down with your hands and begin to straighten your arms as you scoop your chest forward and up. Arch your lower back only as far as it can comfortably go. Move your breastbone up and out, and make sure to widen your shoulders down away from your neck, rather than scrunch your shoulders and neck into each other. Hold for as long as is comfortable, taking long, deep breaths. You may keep your gaze straight ahead, or look up, but be sure to avoid squeezing the back of your neck.

HERBAL REMEDIES

- Mix 1 tablespoon ashwaghanda (Withania somnifera) and 1 pinch each cardamom and saffron with 1 cup hot milk.

- Mix 1 teaspoon ashwaghanda and 1/2 teaspoon each jatamansi (Nordostachys jatamansi) and brahmi (gotu kola) with 1 cup warm milk.

- Saute 1/4 teaspoon nutmeg and 1/2 teaspoon jaggery (brown sugar) in 1 teaspoon ghee.

- Mix 1/2 teaspoon each cardamom and ghee and 'Is tea- -spoon nutmeg with 1 cup warm milk.

AYURVEDA

FIVE-SENSE REMEDIES

- Taste: Emphasize foods and herbs that are sweet, sour, salty, heavy, and oily, but not late in the day. The fall churna is helpful if you also add a little salt and lemon flakes.

- Smell: Sweet, warm aromas, such as basil, orange, rose geranium, and cloves work wonders when inhaled just before bedtime and during sleep.

- Sight: The color green is useful color therapy.

- Hearing: Listen to the late-afternoon raga between four and seven P.M., and the sunset raga as you fall asleep.

- Touch: Apply Brahmi oil to your forehead and navel area before retiring.

IMPORTANT PRECAUTIONS FOR INSOMNIA

Chronic insomnia due to physical illness or emotional imbalance requires professional evaluation and counseling. Medical care should be sought if you experience insomnia for more than 7 consecutive days or if you have a painful medical condition that is keeping you from getting a good night's rest.

INTESTINAL PAIN

Pain is always a sign of a vata imbalance, and -the intestines are the main site for vata dosha. Intestinal pain may be related to an imbalance of agni, the digestive fire, or it may be related to a disturbed peristalsis, the movement that occurs when intestinal muscles contract to move food along the digestive tract. If you press on the ileocecal valve, the point

THE A-Z GUIDE

midway between your navel and your hipbone, and it is tender, it indicates that a specific type of vata is disturbed.

Also see Indigestion for general measures to take for indigestion, and Pain.

AYURVEDIC SELF-CARE

If you are prone to intestinal pain, be sure to follow the appropriate Daily Lifestyle Regimen, paying particular attention to the eating habits and dietary recommendations. Yoga is helpful, and the yoga position called Downward Dog is especially effective.

HERBAL REMEDIES

Choose one of the following:

- Combine 5 parts shatavari (Asparagus racemosus), 3 parts guduchi (Tinospora cordifolia), and 2 parts kama dudha; take 1/4 teaspoon of this mixture with 1 cup warm water, following both lunch and dinner if your pain is very severe.

- Take 1/2 teaspoon amla with 1/4 cup warm water before bedtime.

FIVE-SENSE THERAPIES

- Taste: Sweet, sour, and salty tastes calm vata, so they should be emphasized if you have intestinal pain. The winter churna is the one for you.

- Smell: Sweet, warm smells such as basil, orange, and rose will help ease pain.

- Sight: Blue-green color therapy is recommended.

- Hearing: Listen to the midday raga between the hours of one and four P.M.

- Touch: For 2 weeks apply Bhringhraj oil to the point over your ileocecal valve before retiring.

IMPORTANT PRECAUTIONS FOR INTESTINAL PAIN

Seek medical care if: you experience intestinal pain for more than 3 consecutive days, or the pain is accompanied by fever, nausea, or dizziness.

MENOPAUSE SYMPTOMS

Menopause affects women between the ages of forty-five and fifty-five as their hormone production shifts. You know you have reached menopause only after the fact—menopause actually occurs after the last menstrual period. It's the perimenopause, the time before menopause finally happens, that usually brings characteristic symptoms of hot flashes, mood swings, changes in libido, and insomnia.

Ayurveda considers menopause to be a tri-doshic condition; that is, all three doshas are involved. It begins as a vata imbalance that shakes up pitta and consequently dries kapha. Menopause is one of those life-changing transitions that Mother Nature bestows upon women. It is a change that takes you from the summer, or pitta, time of life (with its ambitions and worldly business) into the fall and winter, or vata time, which can be a tunnel of self-discovery. It is ironic that this is the time women need to learn to accept the ceaseless flow of change in life, just at the time that they experience the cessation of their own menstrual flow.

As you may imagine, this is a challenging phase of life to be in. From my clinical and personal observation, no two women go through it the same way. Some women breeze through. Others suffer severely. Even women who have lived healthy, holistic lives have a wide range of reactions. The Ayurvedic way of going through menopause involves understanding yourself from the doshic perspective, understanding life's cycles, and accepting this time of your life as a powerful challenge with a myriad of influences. Take time out for rest, silence, yoga, breathing, self-massage, nature walks, and—most important -love and understanding.

Also see Confusion, Poor Concentration, and Forgetfulness, Insomnia, and Mood Swings.

AYURVEDIC SELF-CARE

Following the Daily Lifestyle Regimen to rebalance your doshas will greatly ease your passage through this time of life. Many women find that yoga in general is beneficial, particularly the Lion Pose and the Cobra. In addition you may want to take remedies aimed specifically at menopause symptoms:

HERBAL REMEDIES

Choose one of the following:

- Combine 1/2 teaspoon shatavari (Asparagus racemosus) with vata, pitta, or kapha tea, depending on your imbalance.

- Drink 1/2 teaspoon arjuna (Terminalia arjuna) and 1/8 teaspoon yogaraj in 1 cup boiled milk.

FIVE-SENSE THERAPIES

- Taste: Emphasize sweet, sour, and salty to calm vata; use the winter churna every day.

- Smell: Sweet, warm aromas help ease you through this transition, so use aromatherapy with basil, rose, orange, and sage essential oils.

- Sight: Use violet or indigo color therapy.

- Hearing: Listen to the late-afternoon raga between the hours of four and seven P.M.

- Touch: Apply one drop of warm sesame oil and mild finger pressure to the marma points known as Lohitaksa.

IMPORTANT PRECAUTIONS FOR MENOPAUSE SYMPTOMS

Severe menopause can be a sign of hormone imbalances that should be evaluated and diagnosed by a physician. The mood swings, change in libido, and problems with concentration can cause severe emotional instability. If this occurs, combining holistic and conventional medicine is the most effective approach.

MENSTRUAL CRAMPS AND
PREMENSTRUAL SYNDROME (PMS)

Many women experience some form of discomfort before or during their menstrual period. Cramps, back pain, bloating, swollen breasts, food cravings, acne, mood swings, irritability, and fatigue are some of the symptoms from which you may suffer each month. Premenstrual syndrome (PMS) begins at or after ovulation (usually around the middle of the menstrual cycle) and may continue until the beginning of menstruation. Many women continue to experience symptoms such as cramps during menstruation.

PMS has only recently been recognized by the medical establishment as a valid health disorder (it used to be that it was "all in our heads"). Medical specialists now estimate that PMS affects more than 90 percent of fertile women at some point in their lives. In some women the condition is so severe that it disrupts work and social relationships. Hormonal changes

THE A-Z GUIDE

that happen throughout the menstrual cycle clearly influence PMS, but conventional medicine has a myriad of theories on the exact cause of PMS.

In Ayurveda menstrual difficulties are due to an imbalance in the vata and pitta doshas. Vata symptoms have a nervous-system component such as anxiety, fear, insecurity, fatigue, and an inability to think or speak clearly; they also include painful cramps, because vata is responsible for maintaining and toning your muscles. The pitta aspects of PMS are irritability, anger, aggressiveness, feverishness or feelings of heat in the abdominal area, and food cravings; it also plays a part in abdominal swelling. The strength of your digestive fire also influences menstrual symptoms because if the agni is weak and cannot burn off toxins, your body needs to work much harder to release these poisons during menstrual flow. Sometimes kapha is dragged in as well; symptoms include feelings of heaviness and congestion, water retention, breast swelling and tenderness, and heavy flow. The crisis symptoms may be soothed by the self-care Ayurvedic measures and remedies listed below, but curative treatment usually requires a visit to an experienced Ayurvedic doctor.

AYURVEDIC SELF-CARE

Balancing your doshas by adopting the appropriate Daily Lifestyle Regimen, along with the following measures, may be all you need to diminish problems related to menstruation:

Take a warm bath or curl up with a hot-water bottle. Drink hot herbal teas. Warmth increases your blood flow and can relax your cramped pelvic muscles.

Good nutrition helps. Cut out caffeine, alcohol, and salt from your diet. Caffeine can make you nervous and can worsen insomnia and pain. Alcohol and salt may contribute to menstrual bloating. Some women have also found that limiting dairy products can reduce their symptoms of PMS. Eating light and easily digestible meals (bland, low-fat cooked

AYURVEDA

foods including vegetables, fruit, grains, fish, etc.) throughout the day can also reduce that bloated feeling, as well as contribute to your overall health.

Increase your intake of calcium and magnesium. Women taking calcium suffer less from cramps, and magnesium aids in your body's absorption of calcium.

Exercise can help. Moderate activities such as walking and yoga alleviate menstrual cramps in many women. The Child's Pose is particularly soothing for low-back discomfort and pelvic cramps.

HERBAL REMEDIES

- To ease pain: Take 1 teaspoon shatavari (Asparagus racemosus) and 1/2 teaspoon triphala with 1/2 cup warm water every 4 hours.

- To help balance hormones: Take 1/4 teaspoon each shatavari (Asparagus racemosus) and triphala in 1/2 cup warm water daily.

FIVE-SENSE THERAPIES

- Taste: Sweet, bitter, and sour tastes help ease symptoms before and during menstruation, so emphasize foods and herbs in this category; using the winter churna is an easy way to make sure your diet includes these tastes every day.

- Smell: Use aromatherapy with sweet, cool aromas such   as sandalwood, rose, mint, cinnamon, and jasmine.

- Sight: Use blue-green or violet color therapy.

- Hearing: Listen to the midday, late-afternoon, or sunset raga during the appropriate times of day.

- Touch: Apply one drop of warm sesame oil and mild finger pressure to the marina points known as Lohitaksa.

IMPORTANT PRECAUTIONS FOR MENSTRUAL CRAMPS AND PMS

Seek medical care if there is very severe or unusual pain in the pelvic area or abdomen, particularly if accompanied by fever or unusual vaginal bleeding (heavy, clotted, scanty, or none).

If severe menstrual cramps are not relieved by Ayurvedic remedies, don't give up on Ayurveda. It may still work, so seek the advice of a professional. In addition, evaluation and diagnosis by a gynecology specialist is always useful in the treatment of the severe, chronic menstrual disorders.

MIGRAINE HEADACHES

Migraine is a French word derived from the Latin word hemicrania, which means "pain in half of the head." Unlike a tension headache, this type of headache does usually affect only one side of the head, bringing severe throbbing pain. Migraines consist of two phases. In phase one the blood vessels constrict and the brain receives less blood, leading to an early warning sign called an aura. Most often the aura consists of visual disturbances such as visions of light, bright or geometric shapes and lines, and tunnel vision. Other auras include sensations of a strange taste or odor, tingling, dizziness, slurred speech, ringing in the ears, and weakness in a part of the body. This phase may also include nausea, vomiting, chills, and extreme fatigue. As the next phase occurs, the blood vessels open abnormally wide, which stimulates the nerves in the blood vessel walls. The pain begins and is usually accompanied by extreme fatigue.

AYURVEDA

A migraine may last for hours or days and most often affects women. Such headaches tend to run in families. Migraine may be triggered by hypersensitivity or allergic reactions to foods; if you have persistent migraine headaches, allergies are an important consideration. Also at play may be alcohol, bright lights, loud noises, hormonal fluctuations such as occur with the menstrual cycle, and some drugs.

As is the case with tension headaches, migraines and their treatment differ from dosha to dosha:

- Vata migraine headache: This headache starts on the left side and is associated with other common vata disorders, such as insomnia, constipation, and flatulence. It occurs during the vata time of day (two to six P.M. and two to six A.M.) and is aggravated by vata-aggravating foods: bitter, pungent, astringent, thy, hot, and spicy.

- Pitta migraine headache: This type starts on the right side and is associated with pitta disorders such as heartburn, sensitivity to light, and digestive upset. It usually occurs in the middle of the night, worsens during the pitta time of day (ten A.M. to two P.M. and ten P.M. to two A.M.) and improves at night.

- Kapha migraine headache: This headache is usually caused by ama in the form of mucus and is therefore described as sinus headache. Your migraine is of this type if, when you bend over from the waist, the headache feels worse.

AYURVEDIC SELF-CARE

Migraine headache can be so severe that home care measures (and most conventional medicines) don't offer much help. Ayurvedic remedies prescribed by a professional are the best source of relief and prevention. However, following the Daily Lifestyle Regimen to balance your doshas may help minimize migraines. The yoga positions recommended in the section on Tension Headaches may also bring some relief. You may also want to try one or more of the following:

Biofeedback teaches you how to warm your hands by increasing the blood flow to them. This appears to be effective in relieving migraine headaches for some people.

Try to discover what foods might trigger your migraine—several foods have been implicated, including chocolate, nuts, coffee, cheese, citrus fruits, and alcohol. Vata headache is frequently caused by indigestible food combinations, in particular combining milk with yogurt, bananas, or fish.

Repression of natural urges and emotions is one of the most common causes of toxic accumulation and disease. This is especially relevant for migraine because a type of nervous tissue called majja produces tears as a waste product. It is extremely important therefore that you explore any emotions you feel may be trapped inside you.

HERBAL REMEDIES

Start with the tri-doshic remedy (for all doshas), and if that is not effective, use one of the remedies for specific doshas.

- For all doshas: Combine 2 parts brahmi (gotu kola) with 4 parts of either ashwaghanda (Withania somnifera) or shatavari (Asparagus racemosus); take 1/8 teaspoon of this mixture in 1/2 cup boiled milk or water. You may also combine 1 teaspoon vacha (calamus) with enough warm water to make a thick paste and apply to the forehead until the headache is relieved. You may also cut onions to stimulate crying; tears release toxic accumulations in your eyes, sinuses, and brain.

AYURVEDA

- For vata and kapha: Combine 1 teaspoon cinnamon with enough ghee to make a paste and apply to forehead until the headache is relieved.

- For vata and pitta: At onset of symptoms, take one ripe banana blended with 2 cardamom seeds and 1 teaspoon ghee. Repeat, if necessary, every 8 hours.

FIVE-SENSE THERAPIES

- Taste: Vatta and pitta tiypes should emphasize sweet and bitter tastes, while kapha types benefit from pungent taste at this time.

- Smell: Use the aromatherapy tailored to your dosha; for example vata types do well with sweet, warm aromas; pittas with sweet, cool aromas; and kaphas are helped by spicy, warm aromas.

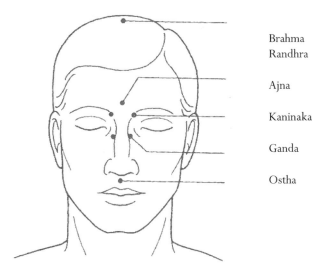

Brahma
Randhra

Ajna

Kaninaka

Ganda

Ostha

The marma points for migraine headache: Brahma Randhra, Ajna Shanka, Kaninaka, Ganda, and Ostha.

- Sight: Use yellow-green color therapy for vata; blue for pitta; and red for kapha.

- Hearing: Listen to ragas during the appropriate hours of the day, depending on your dosha: Vata should listen to the noon or late-afternoon ragas; pitta to the mid-morning raga; and kapha to the sunset raga.

- Touch: Apply one drop of warm sesame oil to the marma points, massaging gently in a clockwise motion.

IMPORTANT PRECAUTIONS FOR MIGRAINE HEADACHES

If your headaches persist despite Ayurvedic treatment, consult your physician; symptoms may be associated with a serious medical condition.

MOOD SWINGS AND IRRITABILITY

One minute you're up, the next you're down. Today the world looks rosy and anything is possible, yesterday your personal sky was full of ominous clouds. Your child can sometimes be an angel and at other times seems possessed by the devil. Uncle Ted was a lamb last week; today he's a cranky old man. Mood swings don't miss any part of the population—young, old, women, and men are all affected.

There have been many explanations proposed for such pendulum-like behavior. From allergies to heredity, they all seem plausible. In Ayurveda an imbalance among all three doshas is considered to be the underlying cause. The body is unable to stabilize and harmonize the daily wear and tear of environmental influences. Vata speeds up, going too fast, and is not able to turn on the digestive fire of pitta. Kapha steps in and tries to

AYURVEDA

stabilize the doshas, but everything may get stuck, creating a "beehive stuck in the mud." The Ayurvedic point of view teaches that you must respect the interactive nature of the body and the emotions, diet, and habits known as addictions. Through this understanding and the use of Ayurvedic practices and remedies, you may be able to even out distressingly dramatic mood swings.

Also see Depression, Menopause Symptoms, and Menstrual Cramps and Premenstrual Syndrome.

AYURVEDIC SELF-CARE

Adopting the appropriate Daily Lifestyle Regimen will help rebalance your doshas and your emotions; be sure to do your yoga Sun Salutations and alternate-nostril breathing faithfully. In addition you may try the following specific remedies on a daily basis, and particularly when a bad mood strikes.

HERBAL REMEDIES

- Drink warm milk combined with 1 teaspoon jatamansi (Nordostachys jatamansi) and 1/2 teaspoon each yogaraj and triphala.

- Eat 2 dates.

FIVE-SENSE THERAPIES

- Taste: Favor sweet, sour, and salty foods and herbs, such as those contained in winter churna.

- Smell: Sweet, warm aromas such as jasmine, rose, and sage help stabilize moods.

- Sight: Color therapy using blue-green or violet may be helpful.

- Hearing: Listen to the sunrise, midmorning, and sunset ragas during the appropriate times of day.

- Touch: In addition to the daily sesame oil massage, massage your ears twice a day. Also massage the Ajna shanka marma point for 60 seconds a day, using firm pressure and a clockwise motion.

IMPORTANT PRECAUTIONS FOR MOOD SWINGS AND IRRITABILITY

If you are presently taking medication, or are under medical treatment for a mood disorder, it is essential to consult your health care practitioner before administering Ayurvedic remedics. If your emotions swing dramatically, be sure to seek medical or psychological help.

MOTION SICKNESS

Motion sickness can occur in a car, boat, or airplane. Mild cases of motion sickness may involve queasiness and/or mild headache. More severe cases entail pallor, heavy sweating, vomiting, and an overall feeling of distress.

This annoying malady is the result of a vata imbalance. Ayurveda can help you minimize the risk of motion sickness as well as restore health after an attack.

AYURVEDIC SELF-CARE

A good general tip is to position yourself defensively during travel. In a car you are less likely to get sick in the front than in the backseat. On a boat stay above deck and to the forward end, where there is less bouncing. And in a plane, get a seat over the wing and avoid the tail, where there is more movement.

AYURVEDA

Ayurveda suggests that you clean out your system before going on a trip. Taking 1/4 teaspoon ghee with 1/2 cup warm water on the day before you leave, will help remove accumulated ama, which would complicate a case of motion sickness. An additional precaution would be to take 1/4 teaspoon fresh grated ginger with a pinch of salt about forty minutes before embarking. This strengthens the digestive juices so that your body can better metabolize the travel experience. In addition you can juice three pears and bring it along with you to take in small amounts as you travel.

HERBAL REMEDIES

The best herbal remedy is to mix 1/2 teaspoon each shatavari (Asparagus racemosus) and dry powdered ginger in 1 cup warm water; drink before and during travel, as needed.

FIVE-SENSE THERAPIES

- Taste: If you can eat, emphasize bitter tastes; you can buy bitters in health food and grocery stores.

- Smell: Bring sweet, warm essential oils with you, such as basil, clove, and rose.

- Sight: The color green helps settle down queasiness due to motion.

- Hearing: Do not listen to music during travel.

- Touch: Press the third eye area in a circular motion; press just above the right side of your upper lip, and hold for 60 seconds. Repeat until you feel relief.

IMPORTANT PRECAUTIONS FOR MOTION SICKNESS

THE A-Z GUIDE

As with any condition of vomiting, if the symptom is relentless and you are unable to hold down fluids, you should be evaluated professionally for dehydration; this may occur after 12 to 24 hours in adults and 8 to 12 hours in children.

NAUSEA

See Abdominal Pain, Indigestion, Motion Sickness, and Vomiting.

PAIN

Pain is a sensation in your nerve endings that can range from mild to excruciating. Pain is usually the immediate sign of an injury, but is a late sign of many disease processes, including cancer. In Ayurveda pain is the result of a vata imbalance and is the cardinal sign of blocked energy. The immune system and juices that function as a cleanup squad become impaired. Blocked ama (toxic residue) clogs the channels and eats away at the nerve and bone fiber of vitality.

It is also important to look at the site of the pain and thus its relationship to the doshas. For example the chest area is where kapha predominates, the abdomen is the pitta area, and the lower intestines and the reproductive organs are principally vata in nature. Pain is most effectively treated if you work on several levels at once: in the site, in the dosha, and in the system, and if you adhere to the appropriate Daily Lifestyle Regimen. Once the pain has subsided, you need to follow up with weekly purification and regenerative practices to help your mind-body heal all aspects of the pain, not just the ones you can feel.

For pain in a particular area of the body, also see Abdominal Pain, Back and Neck Problems, Migraine Headaches, Tension Headaches, Intestinal Pain, Menstrual Cramps, or other conditions that cause pain.

AYURVEDA

AYURVEDIC SELF-CARE

There are several specific remedies that can be incorporated into your Daily Lifestyle Regimen to help relieve generalized pain.

HERBAL REMEDIES

Either one of the following should provide relief:

- Combine 1/4 teaspoon nutmeg, 1/2 teaspoon jaggery (brown sugar), and 1 teaspoon ghee; place a small amount of this mixture in your mouth and allow to dissolve slowly.

- Take 1/2 to 1 teaspoon of the following individually, with 1 cup warm water or milk, or 1 teaspoon ghee; or combine several to suit your taste: calamus root, nutmeg, fennel, cinnamon, cardamom, brahmi (gotu kola), chamomile, cloves, comfrey.

FIVE-SENSE THERAPIES

- Taste: Favor sweet, sour, and salty foods and herbs; the winter churna will provide these tastes in the correct proportions. Add bitter-tasting foods if inflammation accompanies the pain.

- Smell: Sweet, warm aromas such as sage, clove, rose, and orange soothe pain.

- Sight: Blue-green or yellow-green color therapy is helpful.

- Hearing: Listen to the midmorning raga between the hours of ten and one P.M.

- Touch: Apply Brahmi oil for abdominal pain, and massage gently in a clockwise motion.

IMPORTANT PRECAUTIONS FOR PAIN

Pain is a sign your body is in a disease process. If pain persists for three or more days, you should seek a medical diagnosis before continuing with self-care approaches.

PHOBIAS

A phobia is an intense fear of a particular object or situation. This type of fear is usually way out of proportion to the real risk. Almost anything can be the target of a phobia—snakes, heights, spiders, crowds, blood, open spaces, enclosed spaces, public speaking or performing.

The Ayurvedic view sees a phobia as a toxicity in the mind that has developed as a result of the dosha moving in the wrong direction. Usually vata dosha is involved. Fear is the basic emotion linked with a vata imbalance and is common to people with a vata constitution. Phobias are said to be related to a phenomenon in which a person has an association or memory of the phobic object with an unpleasant or life-threatening event. A lifestyle regimen that balances vata is the cornerstone for dealing with phobias; hypnosis may be helpful as well.

AYURVEDIC SELF-CARE

There are several specific remedies that you may incorporate into your Daily Lifestyle Regimen.

HERBAL REMEDIES

- The primary herbal remedy for phobia is ashwagandha ghee. Prepare the ghee by combining 1 part ashwagandha with 16 parts water; boil until 1/4 of the original quantity remains. Add an equal amount of ghee and cook slowly until all the water is gone. Inhale 2 drops into each nostril twice a day, and take 1 teaspoon orally at bedtime. Take this remedy to relieve phobia and as a preventive measure.

- You may also drink fennel-carrot juice; extract the juice of 6 stems of fennel and 2 carrots, and take 3 ounces of this mixture daily. You may also sniff pure fennel juice; put 1 drop into each nostril twice a day.

- Brahmi ghee, sniffed two to three times a day, is also helpful; or you may mix 1 teaspoon Brahmi ghee with warm water and drink it daily. To make Brahmi ghee, add 2 drops Brahmi oil or gotu kola extract to 1/4 cup ghee.

FIVE-SENSE THERAPIES

- Taste: Emphasize sweet, sour, salty foods and oils such as olive, canola, and sunflower. The winter churna is also recommended.

- Smell: Use aromatherapy with sweet, warm aromas including clary sage, orange, and basil.

- Sight: Violet color therapy calms phobic feelings.

- Hearing: Listen to the late-afternoon raga between the hours of four and seven P.M.

- Touch: Daily abhyanga is helpful.

IMPORTANT PRECAUTIONS FOR PHOBIAS

If you feel that your phobia is preventing you from living a normal everyday life, you should seek psychological help from a professional.

THE A-Z GUIDE

PROCRASTINATION

Procrastination flips the old adage, "never put off until tomorrow what you can do today." If you're a constant postponer, putting off tasks until tomorrow, and tomorrow and tomorrow, you have a classic kapha imbalance. Your overwhelming sense of heaviness and lethargy leads to an underwhelming loss of motivation. However, kapha does not break down by itself—rather, all three doshas act together to get to the point where kapha immobilizes you. For example pittas might set impossibly high goals and standards for themselves and this perfectionism stops them from starting for fear of failure. Or the task you are avoiding may be unpleasant—clean up your room or your desk, confront a wrongdoer, reorganize your files—and delay temporarily lessens the tension of facing the inevitable.

AYURVEDIC SELF-CARE

To tackle this stubborn problem, you need to use Ayurvedic technology to wake up, calm down, and motivate your system to get that task done with pleasure and excitement. Use aromatherapy to calm the mind, and kapha tea and hot, light foods to stimulate the mind-body physiology and to lift and lighten the kapha dosha through physical activity, even if it is only a ten-minute walk. The following specific remedies may be incorporated into your Daily Lifestyle Regimen.

HERBAL REMEDIES

- For female procrastinators: Combine 1 part trikatu and 2 parts each saraswati and shatavari (Asparagus racemosus); take 1 teaspoon of this mixture mixed with 1/2 cup warm milk twice a day.

- For male procrastinators: Combine 1 part trikatu and 1 part each triphala and ashwaghanda (Withania somnifera); take 1 teaspoon of this mixture mixed with 1/2 cup warm milk twice a day.

AYURVEDA

FIVE SENSE THERAPIES

- Taste: Emphasize pungent, bitter, astringent tastes; the spring churna supplies these. Also eat hot, light foods.

- Smell: Use sweet, warm essential oils such as basil, orange, clove, and rose.

- Sight: Red-orange color therapy is stimulating.

- Hearing: Listen to the sunset raga between seven and ten P.M.

- Touch: Twice a day, give yourself a facial massage using Mahagenesh oil, paying particular attention to the front and back of your ears, the point where your jawbone meets the ears, and the point midway between your lower lip and chin.

IMPORTANT PRECAUTIONS FOR PROCRASTINATION

This condition could be a sign of depression, so if procrastination persists and is affecting your everyday life, consult a mental health professional.

PROSTATE PROBLEMS

As men grow older, they tend to have problems with the prostate, the walnut-sized gland that produces the fluid that carries sperm. The prostate lies close to the bladder, where urine is stored, and surrounds the urethra, the tube through which urine leaves the body.

Prostatitis is an inflammation and swelling of this gland. The symptoms of acute inflammation are an urge to urinate frequently, a burning sensation during urination, difficulty starting to urinate; fever, weakness, and pain in the area of the prostate which may spread to the genitals, pelvis, or farther up the back. It may feel as though there is a lump in the rectum. Acute prostatitis is often due to a bacterial infection. Chronic inflammation may be due to benign enlargement of the prostate, which is common among older men; chronic inflammation sometimes also occurs after an infection; symptoms are milder but return and linger. The chronic form of this condition may also develop when there is no bacterial infection.

Conventional medicine treats prostatitis with antibiotics (in very acute cases, high-dose intravenous antibiotics are prescribed), but finds chronic prostatitis notoriously difficult to treat. Other medications may be used to relax the urethra, and anti-inflammatory drugs to ease the pain.

In Ayurveda prostatitis is considered to be a pitta disorder in a vata area of the body. Pitta-type prostatitis is characterized by an inflamed bladder and a burning sensation during urination; vata-type is characterized by spasms in the urethra. Ayurveda can help both acute and chronic prostatitis, but be sure to see a health professional before trying home care. The bacteria involved are sometimes particularly dangerous, and the symptoms may also indicate prostate cancer, a common disease in older men.

AYURVEDIC SELF-CARE

Following a Daily Lifestyle Regimen to balance your doshas will help heal an existing episode of prostatitis and reduce the chance of a recurrence. Yoga is also said to be helpful. In addition be sure to . . .

- Drink large amounts of fluids to dilute urine and help

- Wash out the bacteria. Avoid coffee, black tea, and highly seasoned foods, which may cause further irritation.

- Get plenty of rest because as with any acute infection, this helps the body direct its forces toward healing.

- Prevent the prostatic fluid from accumulating and worsening the inflammation by ejaculating every day or every other day. However, during an acute attack you should rest the prostate by avoiding ejaculation and sexual stimulation.

- Do "Kegel" exercises, which may also help in chronic inflammation. To do the exercise, begin by learning to isolate the muscles used to stop and start the flow of urine. Most people find it easier to do this if they begin to urinate and then consciously try to stop the flow. It's likely that you will instinctively tighten the right muscles; these are the same muscles you use to stop a bowel movement or to prevent passing gas. Alternately relax and contract these muscles several times until you can comfortably start and stop urinating. Hold each contraction for a few seconds and then release. Fortunately once you are familiar with the muscles being toned, you don't need to be urinating in order to do the exercises. Since they are an invisible, isometric contraction and relaxation of internal muscles, you can do them almost anytime, anywhere. Do one hundred Kegels each day to encourage the prostate gland to empty its fluid. Alternatively you may have the prostate massaged by a health professional.

HERBAL REMEDIES

- For all types: Drink lemongrass tea every day; take 1/8 teaspoon gokshura (Tribulis terrestris) and 1/2 teaspoon ashwaghanda (Withania somnifera) twice a day for 3 weeks.

- For vata-type prostatitis, which is characterized by spasms of the urethra: Take 3 capsules of saw palmetto daily.

FIVE-SENSE THERAPIES

- Taste: Emphasize sweet, bitter, and astringent tastes found, for example, in the summer churna.

- Smell: Use aromatherapy with sweet, warm aromas such as cloves, basil, and rose.

- Sight: Green color therapy helps with this condition.

- Hearing: Listen to the sunrise and midday ragas during the appropriate times of day.

- Touch: Gently apply Mahanarayan oil (a medicinal oil commonly used for musculoskeletal problems) to the lower back along the five lumbar vertebrae.

IMPORTANT PRECAUTIONS FOR PROSTATE PROBLEMS

Prostate problems need to be evaluated by a physician. Medical care should also be sought if there is pain or swelling in the testicles, in the prostate, or in the surrounding area; if you have had a sexually transmitted disease; if you have trouble starting or maintaining urination, have a weak urine stream, or if you have a discharge from the urethra.

SINUS PROBLEMS (SINUSITIS)

Sinusitis is a swelling of the sinus cavities, the open spaces in your skull above the eyes, within the nose, and inside the cheekbones. During a cold or allergic reaction (such as hay fever, a food reaction, or sensitivity to environmental irritants), the mucous membrane lining the sinus may become swollen. This blocks off the opening leading from the sinus to the nose, causing pressure, pain, congestion, headache, tenderness, or a sense of heaviness behind the eyes and nose, and fever. Other conditions that may cause sinus problems are dental infection and a change in atmosphere (such as air travel or scuba diving).

AYURVEDA

Sinusitis may be mild or severe, acute, chronic, or recurring. When the sinuses become overwhelmed with a bacterial infection, symptoms worsen and there may be a pus-filled discharge from the nose. Sinusitis may affect only one side of the head, or both. Western medicine treats sinus infections with decongestants, pain medication, antibiotics, and, in severe and recurrent cases, surgical drainage.

Ayurveda considers sinus problems to be a sign of severe vata-kapha imbalance. The sinuses have dried up and fill up with debris and mucus. This is a difficult imbalance and requires patience in treating it. Ayurvedic measures and remedies aim to treat the underlying cause—a weak digestive fire.

For additional information also see sections on Colds and Flu, Hay Fever, and Tension Headaches.

AYURVEDIC SELF-CARE

Be sure to follow the Daily Lifestyle Regimen to balance your doshas. The yoga Sun Salutation and Lion Pose are particularly helpful for sinusitis. Also remember to. .

- Take it easy and get rest, especially if the sinusitis is severe.

- Use a vaporizer, humidifier, or bowl of steaming water to loosen mucus and relieve sinus congestion. Wet, hot compresses applied to the painful area may also be soothing.

- Drink plenty of fluids to help liquify mucous secretions.

- As with all infections and allergies, take 2,000 to 3,000 milligrams (2 to 3 grams) vitamin C every day, in divided doses.

THE A-Z GUIDE

HERBAL REMEDIES

Choose one of the following, depending on the predominant doshic imbalance:

- For vata sinus problems, characterized by dizziness; dry, stuffed-up - sinuses; ringing in the ears; and throbbing pain that gets worse with movement: Combine 1/2 teaspoon triphala with 1/4 teaspoon guggul (Commiphora mukul); take twice a day with 1/2 cup warm water, or as needed. In addition you may make a paste of ginger and ghee and apply to the forehead for 20 minutes, until the pain subsides.

- For pitta sinus problems, characterized by tenderness, fever, and green or yellow mucus: Combine 1/2 teaspoon osha, 1/2 teaspoon echinacea, and 1/2 teaspoon guduchi (Tinospora cordifolia); take twice daily with 1/2 cup warm water, or as needed.

- For kapha sinus problems, characterized by dull, aching pain; a sense of heaviness, and thick white discharge: Combine 1/4 teaspoon vacha (calamus) with 1 teaspoon sitopladi; take twice a day with 1/2 cup warm water, or as needed. You may also make a paste of calamus root and water and apply to the cheekbones twice a day. Leave it on for 20 minutes.

- Nasaya (nasal-passage lubrication, with herbs is also helpful. Try sniffing a mixture of 1 drop turmeric extract and 1 teaspoon ghee three or four times a day. If your sinus problems are chronic, do "super nasaya"—inhale 2 drops fresh ginger juice into each nostril. Beware: This will burn and bring tears to your eyes; however, the pain will disappear in 60 seconds and your mind will feel wonderfully clear.

AYURVEDA

FIVE-SENSE THERAPIES

- Taste: Eat predominantly sweet, sour, and salty foods and spices; use the winter churna every day.

- Smell: Aromatherapy using warm, spicy smells such as cedar, eucalyptus, pine, cinnamon, and myrrh help clear up sinus problems.

- Sight: Red and yellow are the colors of choice for color therapy.

- Hearing: Listen to the sunrise, midday, and sunset ragas during the appropriate times of day.

- Touch: Using sesame oil, perform a facial massage, using gentle to firm pressure on the area where you feel pain. Or use eucalyptus oil mixed with sesame oil on the marma points.

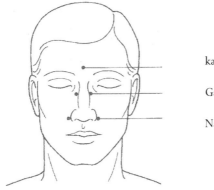

kaninaka

Ganda

Nasa

IMPORTANT PRECAUTIONS FOR SINUS PROBLEMS

Seek medical care if the sinus pain is severe; if there is high fever or a smelly discharge; or if there is an infection that doesn't improve with Ayurvedic care or remedies in 48 hours.

SKIN, DRYNESS AND WRINKLES

These conditions are associated with aging, but dry, tight-feeling, and even itchy skin can appear at any age. Most wrinkles are traceable to overexposure to the sun, but dehydrated, poorly lubricated skin lets wrinkles take hold and exaggerates their appearance. Skin troubles of this type are due to an imbalance in vata, the dry, windy dosha. Dry, flaky, or scaly skin is a reflection of the internal condition—a dry, nervous electrical system. Ayurveda offers both internal and external solutions.

Also see Dermatitis/Eczema and Skin Rash/Hives.

AYURVEDIC SELF-CARE

Follow the Daily Lifestyle Regimen appropriate for balancing your doshas. Sesame oil massage (abhyanga) is a wonderful external and internal lubricant that softens your skin and works to correct the underlying vata imbalance as well.

AYURVEDA

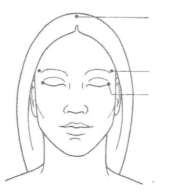

Brahma Randhra

Shankha

Adanga

The marma points for dry skin and wrinkles: Brahma Randhra, Shankha, and Adanga.

HERBAL REMEDIES

- Mix together 1 teaspoon brahmi (gotu kola) and 1 tablespoon ghee; apply this brahmi ghee to the dry areas three times a day.

- Combine the juice of 2 carrots with the juice of 1 bunch of parsley and drink 4 to 6 ounces three times a week.

- Combine 1 part each triphala and yogaraj with 2 parts shatavari (Asparagus racemosus); take 1/2 teaspoon every other day in 1/2 cup warm water.

FIVE-SENSE THERAPIES

- Taste: Emphasize sweet, sour, and salty tastes in your food and herbs; use the winter churna every day.

- Smell: Sweet, cool aromas such as jasmine, mint, and sandalwood are recommended.

THE A-Z GUIDE

- Sight: Blue-green and yellow-orange color therapy is good for dry skin.

- Hearing: Listen to the midday and sunset ragas at the appropriate times of day.

- Touch: Give yourself a daily facial massage with warm sesame oil, pressing your fingertips across your forehead and massaging diagonally from your chin to your eyes. Applying gentle pressure to the marma points helps smooth wrinkles and lubricates dry skin.

IMPORTANT PRECAUTIONS FOR DRY SKIN

If your dry skin persists or is severe, consult a dermatologist to rule out any internal diseases that could be related.

SKIN RASH/HIVES

Skin rashes in general are a classic pitta disturbance, a sign of a disturbed digestive fire, with redness and swelling, perhaps accompanied by fever and irritability. The rash may be infected and is worsened when exposed to heat and sun. Vata rashes are dry and flaky; this is a nervous disorder and is worsened by dry air and wind.

Kapha rashes are wet and oozing and are worse in the damp and cold.

Hives are large, red, inflamed swellings ("welts") that may suddenly appear anywhere on the skin. Hives may also erupt in the respiratory passages. The welts are intensely itchy and may spread quickly, sometimes running together to create larger patches of raised, angry skin. Their appearance is usually tied to certain foods, particularly fruits, nuts, eggs, and certain shellfish; medicines; insect bites; cold; emotional stress; or a recent systemic streptococcal or viral infection. In Ayurveda hives are considered to be due to a pitta imbalance. The digestive fire is burning with acids, causing overproduction of heat, which erupts via the skin. Acute hives may last only a few hours, a day, or a week, and so are self-limiting. Hives may also be a symptom of a chronic condition, which requires treatment by a health care professional.

Also see Allergies and Dermatitis/Eczema.

AYURVEDIC SELF-CARE

Following the appropriate Daily Lifestyle Regimen will eventually help correct the underlying dosha imbalance. In addition you may find that a cool, damp cloth soothes the irritated skin; however, some rashes grow worse with cold application.

HERBAL REMEDIES

- An all-round skin-rash remedy is to apply turmeric powder directly to the affected area three times a day. Exercise caution, since turmeric can stain.

- For hives, juice together 3 kale leaves, 3 collard leaves, and 2 to 3 large slices of pineapple; this should yield

- 4-6 ounces, which you may drink two to three times a day until the hives subside.

- For hives, combine 1 part each manjistha (Rubia cordifolium), guduchi (Tinospora cordifolia), and yogaraj guggulu; take 1/2 teaspoon of this mixture daily for three weeks, or until the rash has subsided.

THE A-Z GUIDE

FIVE-SENSE THERAPIES

- Taste: Emphasize bitter, astringent, and sweet foods   and herbs, and use the summer churna every day.

- Smell: Cool, sweet scents such as mint, sandalwood, and jasmine help calm inflamed skin.

- Sight: Blue color therapy is also calming to the whole system.

- Hearing: Listen to the midmorning raga between the hours of ten A.M. and one P.M.

- Touch: Apply Neem oil to the affected area.

IMPORTANT PRECAUTIONS FOR SKIN RASHES AND HIVES

Consult a physician if there is severe swelling, if hives appear on the mouth or tongue, or if you have trouble breathing. Hives that last for more than a month may indicate internal disease and require professional evaluation.

SORE THROAT

A sore throast can mean many things, most of which are not serious and heal on their own. Ayurveda considers the throat to be a very important bridge between the heart and the mind. The throat is a vata site, and any kind of sore throat indicates a blockage of vata energy. A vata imbalance can express itself by affecting the action responsible for moving things upward; this dries out the natural lubrication, which in itself can cause symptoms of a sore throat, as well as render the throat tissue vulnerable to infection with viruses and bacteria.

AYURVEDA

In this section we provide some general tips and remedies for sore throats. Also see Allergies, Colds and Flu, and Hoarseness for more specific remedies.

AYURVEDIC SELF-CARE

Drink plenty of fluids to lubricate the throat.

Increase the humidity of the air with a humidifier or vaporizer.

Gargling with warm salt water (a pinch of salt dissolved in 6 ounces chlorine-free water), or drinking hot lemonade sweetened with honey, may soothe a sore throat and flush away mucus, viruses, and bacteria.

HERBAL REMEDIES

- Combine 1/2 teaspoon each turmeric and salt; mix in 1 cup warm water and use to gargle twice a day.

- Combine 1/2 teaspoon each cinnamon and licorice with 1 teaspoon honey; place a small amount of this mixture in your mouth and allow to dissolve slowly.

- Combine 1 teaspoon sandalwood and 1/2 teaspoon each powdered ginger and turmeric; mix in 1 cup warm water and gargle twice daily.

IMPORTANT PRECAUTIONS FOR SORE THROAT

Seek medical care if: the pain is severe; swallowing is very difficult; there is a lot of saliva and drooling; there is difficulty breathing; the sore throat is accompanied by fever and doesn't improve in forty-eight hours with Ayurvedic treatment; or a strep culture is needed for public health reasons.

THE A-Z GUIDE

SWOLLEN GLANDS

The term swollen glands usually refers to swollen lymph glands. Lymph glands are part of the lymphatic system, which in turn is part of your immune defense system. So when lymph glands act up and become swollen, it means something is amiss and the immune system is turned on. Enlarged glands in the neck usually accompany sore throats or ear infections; glands in the groin may swell when you have an infection in the genital region, legs, or possibly the feet. Often glands are enlarged even when there's no obvious infection.

In Ayurveda the lymph system is looked upon as part of the body's kapha structures and functions. Since the immune system is really part of your ever-fluctuating nervous system, a stressed, fatigued nervous system may announce itself as a tender, swollen response of your lymph glands.

Also see Colds and Flu and Earaches.

AYURVEDIC SELF-CARE

The following specific remedies may be incorporated into your Daily Lifestyle Regimen.

HERBAL REMEDIES

- Combine 1 part each triphala and sitopladi with 1/2 part mahasudarshan; take 1/2 teaspoon mixed with 1/2 cup warm water every 4 hours until symptoms subside.

- Combine 1/2 teaspoon cinnamon, 1/8 teaspoon powdered ginger, and 3 drops eucalyptus oil in 1/2 cup warm water; inhale 3 drops in each nostril four or five times a day for 3 days.

- Steam fresh okra pods for 5 minutes, then juice them along with the steam water; drink once a day until symptoms subside. This is a traditional remedy for many immunity problems.

FIVE-SENSE THERAPIES

- Taste: Make an effort to include pungent, bitter, and astringent tastes in your food and herbs; use the spring churna, which contains these tastes, every day.

- Smell: Use warm, spicy aromas such as eucalyptus, pine, musk, and cedar.

- Sight: Red-orange color therapy is recommended.

- Hearing: Listen to the sunset raga between the hours of seven and ten P.M.

- Touch: Rub Mahagenesh oil into the front and back of your neck and below the left clavicle (collarbone) area.

IMPORTANT PRECAUTIONS FOR SWOLLEN GLANDS

If your glands are red and tender, have been getting larger over a period of three weeks, do not shrink after three days of self-care, or if you have chronic swollen glands, consult a physician to rule out possible serious infection or other diseases.

THE A-Z GUIDE

TENSION HEADACHES

Almost everyone has had a tension headache at one time or another: this symptom is the most common complaint heard in doctors' offices and in day-to-day life. Some people are more prone to headaches, an indication that the symptom represents an individual's way of reacting to some form of stress. In most cases Ayurvedic home care and remedies have much to offer the person who suffers from the occasional mild headache.

You may be experiencing tension due to mental stress from overwork, for example, or due to the mundane stress of everyday life, such as being stuck in congested traffic. A tension headache may also be the result of physical stress, such as too little sleep, a long, tedious drive, or poor posture. Sometimes both mental and physical stresses are involved, as when sitting at a desk or straining at a computer for long periods of time in order to meet a deadline.

A tension headache usually feels like a dull ache with some tightness and tenderness at the temples, around the forehead, or where the skull meets the neck. It is a common vata disorder, but the symptoms will vary depending upon the predominant dosha of the person (and so will the specific remedy):

Vata-type headache: You have this type of headache if the pain starts in the evening and is throbbing, cutting, acute, and is accompanied by ringing in the ears, dizziness, low backache, gas, constipation, disturbed sleep, tension, anxiety, and insecurity.

Pitta-type headache: This type of headache starts in the middle of the day and the pain is pulling, sucking, burning, throbbing, and sharp and may be accompanied by nausea and disturbed sleep, changes in your eyes, dilated blood vessels, stress, anger, impatience, increased heat, hunger, and being critical or judgmental.

AYURVEDA

Kapha-type headache: The kapha headache starts in the early morning or evening and/or when your stomach is empty. The pain is heavy, dull, and mild and may be related to sinus or bronchial congestion.

Also see Allergies, Anxiety and Fear, Electronic Pollution, and Sinus Problems.

AYURVEDIC SELF-CARE

Practicing the Daily Lifestyle Regimen to balance your dosha will leave you at less risk for headache. It's most important to do yoga Sun Salutations daily and to add the Thunderbolt Pose and the Dynamic Spinal ilvist, shown opposite. Meditation is a proven way to manage daily stress. If you are under more than usual stress, try deep breathing and alternate-nostril breathing, which regulate the release of stress hormones. The Progressive Muscle Relaxation technique is also recommended to break the cycle of tension-muscle tightness that often leads to tension headache. Make sure you get enough sleep and rest if the headache makes you tired or is severe. Other steps to alleviate or prevent headache include the following:

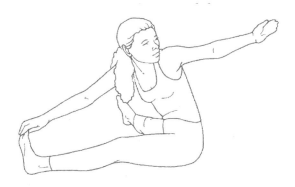

Dynamic Spinal Twist: Sit tall on the floor, with legs straight out in front of you, separated as much as is comfortable. Bring your right hand to your left big toe while stretching your left arm behind you. Both arms should be on a straight line with each other, parallel with the floor. Turn your head

THE A-Z GUIDE

to look behind you at your left hand. Release slowly and twist in the opposite direction. Repeat this set ten or twenty times. Begin slowly, then gradually increase the speed.

Try to determine and relieve the source of stress that is causing the headache. Examples are: poor posture at work, noise, holding the telephone between the ear and shoulder, eyestrain or ill-fitting eyeglasses, and various emotional and social conflicts. Take frequent breaks, periodically look into the distance if you do close work, and get proper work equipment.

Daily sesame oil massage (abhyanga) calms vata, and massaging the scalp, face, neck, shoulders, and back in particular may help relieve a headache.

Look for foods and beverages that may be associated with your headaches. Some people are sensitive to certain foods or combinations; some people get headaches when they do not drink enough fluids; pittas suffer when they skip a meal. Many people have headaches as a withdrawal symptom when they suddenly cut out all coffee—it's better to taper off gradually.

HERBAL REMEDIES

Use the two tri-doshic remedies (for all three doshas), unless your headache is clearly related to a particular dosha.

- For all three doshas: Combine 5 parts shatavari (Asparagus racemosus), 3 parts guduchi (Tinospora cordifolia), 2 parts kama dudha, and 2 parts tikta; take 1/4 teaspoon of this mixture combined with 1/2 teaspoon each ghee and honey twice a day, after eating. Also inhale 3 drops ghee mixed with Brahmi oil in each nostril morning and evening.

- For vata-type headache: Sniff 3 drops calamus oil in each nostril; using an eyedropper, insert 2 to 3 drops warm garlic oil in each ear;

AYURVEDA

rub sesame oil onto the soles of your feet and your forehead. Do this as often as you like.

- For pitta-type headache: Combine 4 parts gotu kola with 3 parts triphala and add 2 parts shatavari (Asparagus racemosus) (women) or ashwaghanda (Withania somnifera) (men); start with Vs teaspoon in 1/2 cup warm water once a day, then gradually increase to 1/2 teaspoon twice a day for two weeks.

- For kapha-type headache: Combine 4 parts triphala, 3 parts sitopladi, and 2 parts trikatu; take 1/2 teaspoon of this mixture with 1/2 cup warm water twice a day.

FIVE-SENSE THERAPIES

- Taste: Sweet, sour, and salty foods, herbs and spices are therapeutic for headache. Try using the winter churna on your foods when headache strikes.

- Smell: Sweet, warm aromas such as clary sage and clove are soothing for a tension headache.

- Sight: Blue-green color therapy is helpful.

- Hearing: Listen to the mid-morning or sunset ragas during the appropriate hours of the day.

- Touch: Apply one drop of warm Brahmi oil to the marma points and gently massage in a circular motion.

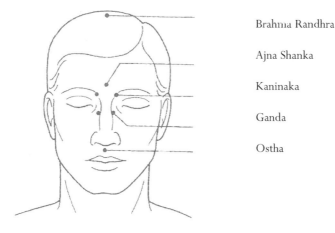

Brahma Randhra

Ajna Shanka

Kaninaka

Ganda

Ostha

The marma points to massage for headache: Brahma Randhra, Ajna Shanka, Kaninaka, Ganda, and Ostha.

IMPORTANT PRECAUTIONS FOR TENSION HEADACHES

Seek medical care when a headache: is unusually severe; lasts more than 3 days; occurs frequently; is steadily worsening; is accompanied by a stiff neck or fever; or occurs after a head injury or after taking a medicine (including birth control pills). Also see a doctor if you have a headache that for the first time is accompanied by migraine symptoms.

ULCER, STOMACH

An ulcer is an erosion of the lining of the stomach or intestine, which is associated with a breakdown of the mucus barrier that normally protects the stomach from powerful digestive acids. In peptic (stomach) ulcers, too much stomach acid, indicating a pitta imbalance, is to blame. When

AYURVEDA

the ulcer occurs in the duodenum (the juncture of the stomach and small intestine), it is due to a vata aggravation.

Oftentimes stress contributes to ulcer formation; smoking also increases the risk and worsens the condition. Other factors include eating irregular meals, alcohol, and many common drugs.

AYURVEDIC SELF-CARE

Follow the appropriate Daily Lifestyle Regimen, paying particular attention to your diet and eating habits, and to stress-reducing practices such as meditation and yoga.

HERBAL REMEDIES

- Mix together 1 teaspoon shatavari (Asparagus racemosus) and 1/2 teaspoon each guduchi (Tinospora cordifolia) and aloe vera gel; take 1 hour before meals.

- Juice together 6 leaves of cabbage, 4 to 5 pineapple slices, and 2 kelp tablets; drink once or twice a week, depending on the severity of your condition.

FIVE-SENSE THERAPIES

- Taste: Emphasize foods and herbs that are bitter, astringent, and sweet; sprinkle the summer churna over your food every day.

- Smell: Sweet, warm aromas soothe the nervous system, so your aromatherapy should consist of essential oils such as sage, rose, and jasmine.

- Sight: The color green helps cool burning ulcers.

THE A-Z GUIDE

- Hearing: Listen to the midday and late-afternoon ragas between the hours of two and six P.M.

- Touch: Apply Brahmi oil to your abdomen and massage in a circular motion.

IMPORTANT PRECAUTIONS FOR STOMACH ULCER

If you suspect you have an ulcer, you should be evaluated by a physician.

VAGINITIS

A woman's vagina and cervix are anatomically designed to secrete fluids. These fluids vary according to the phase of the menstrual cycle, sexual excitement, and pregnancy. A discharge is not necessarily a sign of illness, but you should be aware of any changes in your normal vaginal secretions: the amount, consistency, color, and odor, as well as any other symptoms such as inflammation and itching. Such changes are indications that you have vaginitis, an overgrowth of microorganisms.

Certain conditions can change the balance of normally present microorganisms in the vagina and encourage the overgrowth of one type over another. These include a weakened immune system (for example from stress or overwork), menopause, medications that cause a hormone imbalance, use of chemicals such as birth control products, and others. There are several types of vaginitis, caused by different organisms and characterized by a variety of symptoms.

Yeast infections are so common that you can now buy anti-yeast vaginal creams without a prescription. Also called Candida or monilial infection, a yeast infection of the vagina is characterized by a thick, whitish discharge that may look like cottage cheese and smells like baking bread. Yeast infections can also be maddeningly itchy and the external genital tissues become red and irritated. Yeast may grow out of control after a woman has been treated with a course of antibiotics for a bacterial infection, because the drugs also wipe out vaginal bacteria that kept the normally present yeast in check. Also see Fungus Infection/Candida.

Bacterial infections may be due to a variety of different bacteria. This type of vaginitis is often referred to as nonspecific vaginitis and results in a white or yellow discharge; there may be symptoms similar to cystitis (see Bladder Infections), and lower back pain, cramps, and swollen glands in the groin. Chlamydia and gonorrhea are sexually transmitted bacterial infections that should be identified by means of a professional examination.

Trichomonas infections involve an amoebalike organism and are characterized by a thin, foamy yellowish or greenish discharge that smells offensive. Trichomonas is sexually transmitted and requires a professional examination to identify.

Noninfectious vaginitis may be due to irritation from chemicals (such as douches, diaphragm jelly, or spermicide), sexual activity, or a tampon that has inadvertently been left in. The vagina becomes red and swollen and may produce a discharge to rid the body of the irritation.

Vaginal infections, though annoying, are usually not dangerous. In Ayurveda they are due to a vata imbalance brought about by an aggravated pitta. Ayurvedic home care and remedies can help strengthen the body and speed recovery. The strategy is to cool down the pitta and stabilize the vata influence on the female reproductive organs.

AYURVEDIC SELF-CARE

As you follow the appropriate Daily Lifestyle Regimen, make a special effort to eliminate sweets from your diet during an infection and in general as a preventive measure. Yoga is a wonderful general balancer. The following measures will also help you recover:

THE A-Z GUIDE

Wash your genital area gently and frequently, using mild soap or no soap at all. Pat dry.

If you suspect your vaginitis may be caused by irritation from soap or the fabric of your underwear rather than an infection, avoid the suspected irritant for a time, or switch brands of soap.

Soak in a sitz bath—a bathtub containing six inches of warm water and 1/2 cup vinegar—or douche twice a day with a cleansing douche using 2 tablespoons white vinegar diluted in 1 pint warm water. Vinegar helps change the acid balance of the genital area and helps restore the normal population of organisms.

Plain yogurt may help soothe irritated tissues and restore balance. Apply it directly to the outer tissues, or use a tampon dipped in yogurt and remove in one hour, or dissolve 2 tablespoons yogurt in 1 pint warm water and use as a douche.

Other preventive measures, which may also speed healing, include: avoiding bubble baths, which can irritate delicate genital tissue; avoiding vaginal deodorants; minimizing clothing that encourages overgrowth of organisms by reducing air circulation, such as tight jeans, panty hose, and underwear made from synthetic fabrics; and spending as little time as possible in wet or damp clothing, such as bathing suits or workout clothing.

HERBAL REMEDIES

- Combine 2 teaspoons of turmeric with 1 tablespoon ghee and 1 pint water; use as a vaginal douche, twice a day, morning and evening.

- Mix 2 parts shatavari (Asparagus racemosus) with 1 part each yogaraj and triphala; take 1/2 teaspoon in 1/2 cup warm water twice a day until symptoms subside.

AYURVEDA

FIVE-SENSE THERAPIES

- Taste: The best tastes to treat vaginitis are bitter, astringent, and a small amount of salt.

- Smell: Sweet, warm aromas are recommended, such as sage, rose, and jasmine.

- Sight: Orange, yellow, and green color therapy is recommended.

- Hearing: Listen to the midday and late-afternoon ragas between the hours of One and four P.M. and four and seven P.M.

- Touch: Using a silk glove, give yourself a gentle total-body dry massage every day.

IMPORTANT PRECAUTIONS FOR VAGINITIS

Some infections can be serious and result in infertility. If you have any doubts about the seriousness of your vaginitis, consult a health professional. Medical care should also be sought if: there is significant pelvic or lower abdominal pain; fever is present; you have had a recent new sexual partner; the symptoms occur in a young (prepubescent) girl; there is a heavy discharge that does not improve with Ayurvedic self-care.

VOMITING

Since vata governs movement in the body, the upward motion of vomiting indicates that vata is doing its job. Therefore, according to Ayurveda, in many cases vomiting is the body's own wise response and an important step in healing. So if vomiting occurs and then is immediately over, consider it a positive event! However, if vomiting

THE A-Z GUIDE

persists, it indicates a prolonged health problem, because poison is still trapped inside your body.

Also see Indigestion and Nausea.

HERBAL REMEDIES

- To stop vomiting, drink 1 cup warm water to which you have added 1 teaspoon honey and 1/2 teaspoon each powdered cardamom, fennel, and cloves.

FIVE-SENSE THERAPIES

- Taste: When you are able to eat again, add a little salt and lemon flakes to the summer churna and sprinkle on your food.

- Smell: Sniff sweet, warm, sour aromas such as basil, clove, orange, and rose.

- Sight: The color green is good therapy because it calms pitta and vata.

- Hearing: Listen to raga music composed for the hours between ten A.M. and one P.M.

- Touch: Apply one drop of warm sesame oil and finger pressure to the marma point known as Ostha.

IMPORTANT PRECAUTIONS FOR VOMITING

If vomiting is severe, contains blood, or is persistent, there could be poisoning, infection, or a serious disease, so be sure to call for medical help.

AYURVEDA

WARTS

Warts, also called verrucae, are skin growths related to viruses. Common warts may crop up in the hands, feet, and face; plantar warts are found on the soles of the feet; and venereal warts affect the genitals and surrounding area. Wart viruses are contagious; however, some people appear to be more susceptible than others. Conventional medicine treats these growths with caustic chemicals, electricity, freezing, and surgery. Ayurveda believes warts to be a sign of a breakdown among all three doshas. Vata becomes aggressively imbalanced and infiltrates the other two doshas and the tissues they govern. This invasion leaves tissues vulnerable to viral invasion and overgrowth, including the viruses that cause warts. As with all viral infections, Ayurveda aims to increase the strength of your immune system so that your inner healer can throw off the infection and make the warts fall off.

AYURVEDIC SELF-CARE

The Ayurvedic approach is from the inside out, and from the outside toward your inner physiology. Sometimes hypnosis or the power of suggestion rouses the body's vital force to throw off the warts. Children can be encouraged to say "good-bye" to their warts as they stroke them two or three times every night before bed. Following the appropriate Daily Lifestyle Regimen for your dosha will help restore immune strength. You also need to purify your system and take antiviral herbs. A good general purifier is to drink the juice of half a lemon mixed with warm water every day upon arising. A daily dose of 6 to 8 ounces half-raisin and half-grape juice is a traditional recipe for strengthening the immune system against all infectants, including viruses. Gentle, natural purgatives such as senna are also recommended.

THE A-Z GUIDE

HERBAL REMEDIES

Combine 1 part each manjistha (Rubia cordifolium) and yogaraj guggulu with 1/2 part mahasudarshan; take 1/2 teaspoon in 1/4 cup warm water twice a day. For children, use just a pinch twice a day.

- Combine 1 teaspoon honeysuckle and 1/2 teaspoon forsythia with 1 cup hot water; take this antiviral herbal once a day.

- Combine 1 tablespoon Neem oil with 1/2 teaspoon turmeric; apply with a cotton swab every night before bed. (Be careful, as turmeric will stain.)

FIVE-SENSE THERAPIES

- Taste: Bitter is the taste of choice for getting rid of warts; eat bitter foods and herbs, such as bitter melon, which is a powerful antiviral.

- Smell: Use aromatherapy with essential oils that smell spicy and warm, such as sage, pine, and eucalyptus.

- Sight Yellow-orange color therapy is reputed to help make warts disappear.

- Hearing: Listen to the midday and late-afternoon ragas between the hours of one and four and four and seven P.M.

- Touch: Daily abhyanga using almond oil is recommended.

IMPORTANT PRECAUTIONS FOR WARTS

Seek medical care if the warts are on the genitals; genital warts can be a sign of syphilis and must be examined by a qualified medical professional.

AYURVEDA

WATER RETENTION (BLOATING)

Our bodies are normally 75 percent water, but sometimes it feels more like 99 percent. Many women complain that they particularly retain water just before and during their menstrual periods, but that bogged-down feeling can strike anytime that kapha becomes sluggish. Some people, for example, are bothered by swollen fingers and ankles during hot, humid weather. In Ayurveda maintaining the proper water balance in the body is kapha's job. Kapha becomes congested when vata becomes imbalanced and stops directing traffic. As a result the lungs, heart, kidney, and other tissues clog up. You feel bloated and heavy, inside and out, as your waterlogged tissues expand and hold water instead of circulating it.

AYURVEDIC SELF-CARE

Along with following the appropriate dosha-balancing Daily Lifestyle Regimen, you may find the following remedies helpful in ridding your body of excess water:

HERBAL REMEDIES

- Take 1 teaspoon triphala with 1 cup warm water before bedtime, then add one of the following:

- Make a tea using 1 teaspoon fennel per 1 cup hot water and drink three times a day.

- Combine 1/3 teaspoon each of punarnava (Boerrhavia diffusa), gokshura (Tribulis terrestris), fennel, and sandalwood with 1 cup hot water; drink three times a day.

- Take 1/2 teaspoon punarnava (Boerrhavia diffusa) twice a day with 1 cup water.

- Watermelon juice is an effective and delicious natural diuretic; drink one small glass three times a day when this fruit is in season.

FIVE-SENSE THERAPIES

- Taste: Pungent, bitter, and astringent tastes should be emphasized; the spring churna is an excellent way to introduce these tastes into your everyday diet.

- Smell: Essential oils with spicy, warm aromas help stimulate kapha and regulate water in the body.

- Sight: The color red is also stimulating, and recommended.

- Hearing: Listen to the sunset raga between seven and ten P.M.

IMPORTANT PRECAUTIONS FOR WATER RETENTION

None.

WEIGHT PROBLEMS

In Ayurveda underweight and overweight are signs that the vata, pitta, and kapha systems are out of balance. Both can occur, regardless of how much or how little food you eat, because your intake is not being properly metabolized.

For example overweight is usually a problem for people with predominantly kapha-type constitutions. When this dosha, which is composed of water and earth, is imbalanced, the heavy characteristics of these elements become exaggerated. Pitta types are generally of medium build, but if the digestive fire is too low because they have burned themselves out, food isn't processed properly, and this results in weight

AYURVEDA

gain. For vata types the problem is usually underweight. When vata is imbalanced, the components of the nervous system, the pituitary, the thyroid, and the hypothalamus become overwhelmed or jammed. The neuroelectrical circuits that are the expression of vata energy become deranged, and the system cannot absorb nutrients. However, even vata types can become overweight when imbalanced if they attempt to calm and lubricate their overstimulated and dry nervous systems with sweet, oily foods.

In our practice many people seek help for many other problems, but don't even mention their weight because they have become so discouraged about it. They invariably are pleasantly surprised to find that excess pounds come off naturally. If you have been struggling with your weight for quite some time, you, too, may be feeling hopeless. Perhaps you have counted calories, followed the latest popular diet that promises you'll shed twenty pounds in twenty minutes, and have experienced the terrible sensation of feeling just a little hungry all the time. Or perhaps you've struggled in vain to put some meat on your bones. The Ayurvedic approach to achieving your ideal weight is not just a matter of counting calories and watching the food you eat. It is about getting to know your body and becoming in tune with its rhythms; it means taking a realistic look at your body type and what it can be, and then nourishing it back to natural health.

AYURVEDIC SELF-CARE

Whether you want to lose or gain weight, the strategy is to permanently reset your mind-body's ability to regulate itself by calming the nervous system, enhancing your digestive fires, and regulating the storage of energy and fat.

HERBAL REMEDIES FOR UNDERWEIGHT

- Each month do the Ten-Day Ginger Treatment.

THE A-Z GUIDE

- To deeply calm the nervous system, combine equal parts of jatamansi (Nordostachys jatamansi) and vacha (calamus); take 1/2 teaspoon with 1/2 cup warm water twice a day.

FIVE-SENSE THERAPIES FOR UNDERWEIGHT

- Taste: Sweet, sour, salty tastes should be emphasized; the winter churna is an excellent way to introduce these tastes into your everyday diet.

- Smell: Essential oils with sweet, warm aromas help calm vata and your nervous system, so choose jasmine, sandalwood, basil, cinnamon, and orange scents for your aromatherapy.

- Sight: The color green is also calming, and recommended.

- Hearing: Listen to the midday and late-afternoon ragas during the appropriate hours.

- Touch: Daily sesame oil massage calms and lubricates an overwrought nervous system.

AYURVEDIC SELF-CARE FOR OVERWEIGHT

The specific approach depends on the dosha, but in general you need to follow the Daily Lifestyle Regimen and diet for your constitution while increasing your intake of foods that enhance your digestive fire. These include ginger, papaya, mango, pineapple, bitter melons, and dark, bitter greens.

You also need to reconnect with your inner self and your present life. Ask yourself, how do I feel? What weight do I want to be? Am I hungry for something other than food? If you are not satisfied emotionally or psychologically, you need to look at that—are you using food to fill a void that is best taken care of in other ways? Are you nourishing all your senses? We have found that using therapy that attends to all five senses is a magical approach to weight loss. In addition your body needs relaxation and oxygen—these two nutrients are essential to achieving balance, so be sure to practice yoga, meditation, and pranayama (breathing exercises) daily.

And finally, exercise, exercise, exercise, using the form that is most beneficial for your dosha. Vata types need movement with a gentle pace, such as tai chi, many forms of yoga, and perhaps a light amount of dance aerobics and resistance training (weights). Pittas do best with challenging and vigorous hikes surrounded by green nature and blue skies, and competitive sports. Kaphas require very vigorous activity, such as running, dancing, hiking, swimming, triathalons.

HERBAL REMEDIES FOR OVERWEIGHT

- The following herbal remedy is recommended for all three doshas; its taste leaves something to be desired, but the unpleasantness is worth it because it really works wonders:

- Combine 1 part each chitrak (Plumbago zeylonica), kukti, and trikatu; take 1/2 teaspoon with a mouthful of warm water, swish around your mouth, and swallow. Take this once a day if you are 20 pounds overweight or less; take twice a day if you are more than 20 pounds overweight.

VATA FIVE-SENSE THERAPIES FOR OVERWEIGHT

- Taste: Emphasize bitter, pungent, and astringent tastes, such as those found in the spring churna; also add sweet taste in the form of rice and dates, and a little oil to your foods.

- Smell: Essential oils with sweet, warm aromas help calm vata and your nervous system, so choose jasmine, clove, rose, cinnamon, and orange scents for your aromatherapy.

THE A-Z GUIDE

- Sight: The color yellow-green is recommended.

- Hearing: Listen to the late-afternoon raga between four and seven P.M.

- Touch: Daily full-body oil massage (abhyanga) is essential. Also combine 3 drops rose aromatherapy oil with 2 teaspoons sesame or almond oil and apply this to your wrist and to the back of the head where the skull meets the neck bones (occipital ridge).

PITTA FIVE-SENSE THERAPIES FOR OVERWEIGHT

- Taste: Choose bitter, pungent, and astringent tastes, such as those found in the spring chuma; bitter foods are especially beneficial, such as bitter melon, dark green leafy vegetables, bitter lettuces such as arugula, and tart apples.

- Smell: Essential oils with sweet, cool aromas help stabilize vata, so choose honeysuckle, mint, and jasmine scents for your aromatherapy.

- Sight: The color indigo blue is recommended.

- Hearing: Listen to the midmorning raga between the hours of ten A.M. and one P.M.

- Touch: To stimulate and purify, give yourself a ten-minute garshana (thy) massage every morning using a silk glove.

KAPHA FIVE-SENSE THERAPIES FOR OVERWEIGHT

- Taste: There are many ways to use taste therapy for kaphas. Generally bitter, pungent, and astringent tastes are recommended. These are found in many foods and spices—you can't eat too much ginger in particular—as well as the spring churna, which you can

AYURVEDA

sprinkle on your food every day. Drinking the following peppy juice will burn the pounds away, but admittedly is only for the stout of heart: Mix the juice of 5 large slices of fresh pineapple with the juice of 2 slices of hot peppers, pimentos, or paprika. Also try this herbal remedy: Mix 1 part each turmeric, triphala, and trikatu with 2 parts honey; take 1/2 teaspoon once a day with 1/2 cup warm water.

- Smell: Warm, spicy aromas help stimulate kapha to burn up fat, so use eucalyptus, pine, musk, and sage aromatherapy.

- Sight: The color red is recommended to stimulate sluggish kapha.

- Hearing: Listen to the sunset raga between the hours of seven and ten P.M.

- Touch: Daily dry massage (garshana) using a silk glove is stimulating. You may also make an herbal paste of 1 part millet and 1/2 part each dashmoola and bala (Sida cordifolia) mixed with a little spring water. Rub this vigorously onto your skin wherever you have fatty deposits, then rinse.

THE A-Z GUIDE

GLOSSARY OF TERMS

ABHYANGA (ah-bee-YANG-ah) A massage with oil, usually sesame oil

AGNI (AHG-nee) The digestive fire that helps break down food, feelings, thoughts, and everything you take in through your senses

AMA (AH-mah) Impurities remaining after improper digestion; when ama accumulates in the mind-body, imbalances in your doshas may occur, then symptoms, and eventually disease

ASANA (AH-sah-nah) Yoga pose

AYURVEDA (ah-your-VAY-dah) The science of life and longevity that is a six-thousand-year-old healing tradition from India

CHURNA A combination of powdered herbs and spices

DOSHA (DOH-shah) The governing principle or force responsible for controlling the functions of your mind and body; the three doshas are called vata, pitta, and kapha

GARSHANA (gar-SHAH-nah) A dry massage performed with silk gloves

GHEE (GEE) Clarified butter, used in Ayurveda to lubricate the mind-body and to enhance the effectiveness of herbs and spices

KAPHA (KAH-fah) One of the three doshas; it is composed of water and earth and is responsible for body structure

MARMA (MAR-mah) One of the 108 points on the skin that are stimulated by Ayurvedic massage and yoga

NASAYANA (nah-SAH-yah-nah) Inhaling oil to cleanse and lubricate the nasal passages and sinuses

OJAS (OH-jas) The pure end product of proper digestion

PANCHA KARMA (PAHN-cha-KAR-mah) Cleansing and purifying techniques used in Ayurveda

PITTA (PIT-tah) One of three doshas; it is composed of fire and water and is responsible for metabolism

AYURVEDA

PRAKRUTI (prah-KROO-tee) Your essential nature, as expressed by the proportion of the three doshas you were born with

PRANA (PRAH-nah) The life force, or breath; similar to chi in Chinese medicine

PRANAYAMA (PRAH-nah-YAH-mah) Breathing exercises

RASAYANA (RAH-sah-YAH-nah) Remedies and tonics based on combinations of herbs and spices

TRI-DOSHA (TRY-doh-shah) The three doshas together; often refers to a remedy or practice that stabilizes all three doshas simultaneously

VATA (VAH-tah) One of the three doshas; it is composed of air and space and is responsible for movement

VIKRUTI (veh-KROO-tee) Your current condition; the ratio of your three doshas that fluctuates along with your health

YOGA A practice of movement (asanas) and breathing (pranayama) that dissolves the separation between mind and body; it prepares the practitioner for meditation as well as encourages the nervous system, endocrine system, internal organs, and muscles to function at their optimum level

THE A-Z GUIDE

FURTHER READING

There are many excellent books on Ayurveda for those who wish to delve more deeply into this health system. The following are highly recommended:

Chopra, Deepak. Ageless Body, Timeless Mind: The Quantum Alternative to Growing Old. New York: Harmony Books, 1993.

Creating Health: How to Wake Up the Body's Intelligence. Boston: Houghton-Mifflin, 1991.

Perfect Health. New York: Harmony Books, 1990.

Quantum Healing: Exploring the Frontiers of Mind Body Medicine. New York: Bantam, 1989.

Frawley, David. Ayurvedic Healing: A Comprehensive Guide. Salt Lake City: Passage Press, Morris Publishing, 1989.

Frawley, David, and Vasant Lad. The Yoga of Herbs: An Ayurvedic Guide to Herbal Medicine. Santa Fe: Lotus Press, 1988.

Iyengar, B.K.S. Light on Pranayama. New York: The Crossroad Publishing Company, 1987.

Lad, Usha, and Vasant Lad. Ayurvedic Cooking for Self-Healing. Albuquerque: The Ayurvedic Press, 1994.

Lad, Vasant. Ayurveda: The Science of Self-Healing. Santa Fe: Schocken Press, 1984.

Packard, Candis Cantin. Pocket Guide to Ayurvedic Healing. Freedom, Calif.: The Crossing Press, 1996.

AYURVEDA

Shanbhag, Vivek. A Beginner's Introduction to Ayurvedic Medicine. New Canaan, Conn.: Keats Publishing, 1994.

Sharma, Hari. Freedom from Disease. Toronto: Veda Publishing, 1993.

Svoboda, Robert E. Lessons and Lectures on Ayurveda. Albuquerque: The Ayurvedic Institute, 1984.

Prakruti: Your Ayurvedic Constitution. Albuquerque: Goecom Limited, 1988.

Tiwari, Maya. Ayurveda: A Life of Balance. Rochester, Vt.: Healing Arts Press, 1995. (Ayurvedic nutrition and recipes.)

We also recommend the following books, which are related to the Ayurvedic way of life:

Ackerman, Diane. A Natural History of the Senses. New York: Vintage Books, 1991.

Alexander, C. N., et al. "Transcendental Meditation, Mindfulness, and Longevity: An Experimental Study with the Elderly." Journal of Perspectives in Social Psychology 57 (1989):950-64.

"Transcendental Meditation, Self-Actualization, and Psychological Health: A Conceptual Overview and Statistical Meta-analysis. Journal of Soc. Behay. Perspectives 6 (1991):189-247.

Dileepan, K. N., et al. "Priming of Splenic Lymphocytes After Ingestion of an Ayurvedic Herbal Food Supplement: Evidence for an Immunomodulatory Effect." Biochemistry Archives 6 (1990):267-74.

Eisenberg, D. M., et al. "Unconventional Medicine in the United States: Prevalence, Costs, and Patterns of Use." New England Journal of Medicine, vol. 328, no. 4 (Jan. 28, 1993):250.

Eppley, K., et al. "Differential Effects of Relaxation Techniques on Trait Anxiety: A Meta-Analysis." Journal of Clinical Psychology 45 (1989):957-74.

Lee, J. Y. The Antioxidant and Antiatherogenic Effects of MAK-4 in WHHL Rabbits. Ph.D. Dissertation, the Ohio State University, Columbus, Ohio, 1995.

Misra, N. C., et al. "Antioxidant Adjuvant Therapy Using a Natural Herbal Mixture MAK During Intensive Chemotherapy: Reduction in lbxicity. A Prospective Study of 62 patients." In Proceedings of the Sixteenth International Cancer Congress, edited by R. S. Rao, et al. Bologna, Italy: Monduzzi Editore, 1994, pp. 3,099-102.

Niwa, Y. "Effect of Maharishi-4 and Maharishi-5 on Inflammatory Mediators with Special Reference to Their Free Radical Scavenging Effect." Indian Journal of Clinical Practice 1 (1991):23-27.

Orme-Johnson, D. "Medical Care Utilization and the Transcendental Meditation Program." Psychosomatic Medicine 49 (1987):493-507.

Patel, V., et al. "Reduction of Mouse Lewis Lung Carcinoma (LLC) by M-4 Rasayana." FASEB Journal 4 (1990):A637. Abstract.

Prasad, K. N., et al. "Extract of Maharishi Amrit Kalash-5, an Ayurvedic Herbal Preparation, Induces Differentiation in Neuroblastoma Cells in Culture." Presented at Eighth Biennial Meeting, International Society of Developmental Neuroscience; June 16, 1990, Bar Harbour, Florida.

Sharma, H. M., et al. "Antineoplastic Properties of Dietary Maharishi-4 and Maharishi Amrit Kalash Ayurvedic Food Supplements." European Journal of Pharmacology 183 (1990):193.

"Antineoplastic Properties of Maharishi-4. Against DMBA-induced Mammary Tumors in Rats." Pharmacology and Biochemical Behavior 35 (1990):767-73.

"Improvement in Cardiovascular Risk Factors Through Panchakarma Purification Procedures." J. Res. Educ. Indian Medicine, vol. 12, no. 4 (1993):2-13.

"Maharishi Amrit Kalash (MAK) Prevents Human Platelet Aggregation." Clinical Ter. Cardiovasc 8 (1989):22730.

Sundaram, V., et al. "Increased Resistance of Human LDL to Oxidation in Hyperlipidemic Patients Supplemented with Oral Herbal Mixture MAK." FASEB Journal, vol. 9, no. 3 (1995):A141. Abstract.

Waldschutz, R. "Influence of Maharishi Ayur-Veda Purification Treatment on Physiological and Psychological Health," Erfahrungsheillcunde-Acta medico empirica 11 (1988):720-29.

Wallace, R. K. "Physiological Effects of Transcendental Meditation." Science 167 (1970):1751-54.

Sharma. H. M. "Maharishi Ayur-Veda: An Ancient Health Paradigm in a Modern World." Alternative and Complementary Therapies, Nov.— Dec. 1995, pp. 364-72.

Sharma, H. M., et al. "Letter from New Delhi. Maharishi Ayur-Veda: Modern Insights into Ancient Medicine." Journal of the American Medical Association, vol. 265, no. 20 (May 2229, 1991):2633-37. Also response letters published in vol. 266, no. 13 (Oct. 2, 1991):1769-74.

INDEX

AYURVEDA

THE A-Z GUIDE

Made in the USA
San Bernardino, CA
02 February 2015